Dirty Girl

Dirty Girl

Ditch the Toxins,
Look Great and
Feel FREAKING AMAZING!

WENDIE TRUBOW, MD
and ED LEVITAN, MD

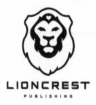

LIONCREST
PUBLISHING

DIRTY GIRL

Ditch the Toxins, Look Great and Feel FREAKING AMAZING!

ISBN   978-1-5445-2236-4   *Hardcover*

       978-1-5445-2235-7   *Paperback*

       978-1-5445-2234-0   *Ebook*

Contents

Introduction

Everybody thinks being dirty is sexy and fun. That it's exciting and titillating. As if it's everything decadent that your mother always warned you about. But I'm here to tell you everybody is wrong. In fact, for me, being a dirty girl was anything *but* fun and exciting.

My life as a dirty girl was one filled with brain fog, stomach bloating, and exhaustion—and none of it came from being hungover. In fact, I didn't intentionally do anything to deserve being the dirty girl I was. I never once replied to a text saying *Wine not?* Nor have I ever flirted my way to the front of a line at a club! Well, *maybe* I did once or twice.

Regardless, some would say I was the poster child for clean living. I didn't eat sugar. I said no to refined carbs. I didn't drink alcohol. I didn't smoke. And I exercised like a fiend. I was doing everything right! So why did I look and feel so wrong? Where was the energy I used to have? The quick wit? Why were all my clothes so tight? Why couldn't I remember my middle name sometimes? Why did the idea of having sex sound about as fun as staring at cement? And somebody, please tell me: Why. Is. My. Hair. *Falling. Out?!?*

Why? Because, after doing some testing, I discovered I was a hot toxic mess.

Which begs the next question: how did that happen?

We're All in This Together

The *how* is grounded in the fact that we live in the twenty-first century. No one really knows how many toxins are in the air we breathe, the foods we eat, the water we drink, or even what's emanating off our clothing and furniture. Which means no one knows how much we're absorbing, breathing, and ingesting on a daily basis.

If the *occasional* toxin were all we were ever exposed to, then most of us would have no problem naturally detoxing it out of our systems. But because the world around us is becoming more and more toxic, we don't just have an occasional toxin that we need to deal with. We have a perpetual onslaught that is straining our systems' ability to metabolize them. On top of that, our lifestyles make it even harder. Prolonged stress, undiagnosed food sensitivities, and even our genetic makeup can hinder how well we detox. And when the body becomes overwhelmed by unresolved stress and sensitivities, it can lose the ability to detox altogether. When that happens, the body just can't keep up. It has no other option but to store the excess toxins in fat, tissues, organs, and sometimes in our bones. After a while, though, even that becomes ineffective, and our bodies start sending signals telling us we need help, that we need to get the toxins out.

I missed those signals for a long time.

Just as you might be, I'm busy. My husband, Ed, and I have a thriving medical practice, Five Journeys. We have four active children and live near extended family, so I'm often involved with activities involving all of them. Of course, I'm also managing our house, cooking, grocery shopping, finding the right supplies for school projects, and on and on and on. You probably get the picture because it's probably very similar to *your* life.

I love most of it—if it weren't for the fact that it feels like I always need to get some laundry done, I'd probably love all of it. And I give it my all. But when the digestive troubles and brain fog got in the way, my all became a little lacking. I even started withdrawing socially because I just didn't have the energy to handle the negative consequences my gut would throw at me after going out to eat. Add in muscle soreness and weakness, and my "all" slipped even more.

When I thought things couldn't get any worse, in late peri-menopause, I found out I was wrong. That's when the hair loss started and I gained nine pounds for no reason....Just what every woman wants, right?

The thing is, I was familiar with all the above symptoms. Usually, they are signs of an imbalanced or toxic body. Not only have I seen numerous patients in that condition, but I've found great success in helping them heal. Through balancing out and detoxifying their bodies, they become the vibrant, happy, and healthy (clean) people they were meant to be. So I thought maybe I should start treating myself the way I'd treat a patient.

You've Got Mold

At Five Journeys, people come to us for a variety of reasons and a full range of symptoms that are similar to mine, and often more extreme. Many have mysterious skin issues or rashes that just won't go away with treatment. Some show signs of anxiety and depression. Hair loss, brittle nails, brain fog, and menstrual aberrations are all very "normal" for the women we see. Meanwhile, the men who come in are usually more concerned with their decreased energy and sex drive.

By the time many of our patients come to us, they have been feeling off-balance or just "out of whack" for a long while, and their primary care doctors haven't been able to figure out why. Or they've been battling a host of symptoms for years and are still looking for the right approach to alleviate them. Being in the Northeast, it's not abnormal for many of our patients to have been previously diagnosed with Lyme disease and, even though they've been treated for it, still be symptomatic. But some of our patients are relatively healthy and are just looking for ways to achieve optimum health.

After checking an extensive list of health indicators for our patients, meaning things like gut health, cardiovascular health markers, and comprehensive nutrient levels, one of the next major things we do is order tests to look for toxins: mycotoxins from mold, environmental toxins, heavy metals, pesticides/glyphosate (weed killer), or all four. So that's what we did with me.

I began with a mold test. And holy sh*t, Batman! I had four strains of mycotoxins (yes, four different kinds of mold toxins) in me, including ochratoxin, which comes from black mold as well as a variety of foods. But that was just the tip of the iceberg. Later testing revealed that heavy metals, pesticides, and a variety of other toxins were having their way with me too. I couldn't believe it at first. I thought I had been doing everything right! Yet somehow the poster child for clean living was more polluted than a toxic waste dump.

I needed to figure out how to clean up my act.

Getting Clean

It might sound crazy, but getting a positive toxicity profile can actually be a good thing. Once you get that data, you are given the power to do something about your health. By following a detox protocol specific to *your* toxic burden load, you can begin to alleviate the symptoms that have been plaguing you and, over time, even reverse them.

In my case, a few months after starting the mold removal program, I realized that my gluten sensitivity wasn't so sensitive. Don't get me wrong: as a person with celiac disease, gluten is never kind to me, and I never, ever, ever eat it on purpose. However, when my body was overburdened by the persistent effort to deal with the toxins, it was not able to handle the slightest exposure to gluten. I would become sick within a half hour of eating a tiny cross-contaminated amount. And, in some of the worst instances, I wouldn't recover for six to eight weeks (once it took three months). During that time, I'd battle brain fog, have diarrhea several times a day, and feel anxious (not to mention the terrible, room-clearing gas). There were times when my gluten reaction was so bad, I could barely work. However, once my mold toxins started coming down, I realized the gluten sensitivity was more tolerable. Not that I ever intentionally indulge in it, but now when there's an accidental exposure, the symptoms are much milder, and they generally go away within twenty-four hours. In fact, I've recently been able to dine outside my home at restaurants that offer gluten-free foods. That may not sound like much to a person who doesn't live with celiac disease. But it's a life-changer for me! I know sometimes those restaurants accidentally have cross-contamination issues. I just couldn't risk an unintended micro-exposure in the past. Now I'm not only willing to brave it, but I am able to recover from it more quickly if I get exposed.

Detox from mold and other toxins almost always has positive effects for our clients. Skin issues clear up, rashes go away, and discomfort is soothed. Irritable bowels become nice and gentle. Energy levels increase, and sexual appetites are suddenly a "thing" again. There is improved brain function and clearer thinking. And one of the biggest prizes for many of the women I see? They're finally able to lose weight.

But Wait! There's More!

After that initial discovery of mold toxins in my body, I bit the bullet and began running a variety of other tests. It turned out that I was one hot toxic mess! There were toxins in my body I'd never even heard of. It almost didn't make sense.

Of course, though, it really does make sense. From an outsider's perspective, it might even look like someone had stacked the deck against me to ensure I became toxic. We'll explain in

Chapter 1 why toxicity was almost predetermined for me (and might be for you). Then, in Chapter 2, we'll discuss stress. My life had been a pretty stressful one, particularly as an adult. The thing to remember about stress is that it can shut down normal activities, which knocks certain systems out of balance in your body. In particular, it takes so much of your body's reserves and energy that your liver and natural detoxification pathways just cannot work correctly to eliminate toxins.

And toxins are everywhere! Chapters 3 through 5 discuss the myriad potential avenues toxins use to sneak into our bodies. We ingest them directly in our food and water. We absorb them into our skin from our body care and beauty products as well as from our clothing and furniture. We also breathe them in, whether it's from breathing the polluted air outside or air contaminated by off-gassing household goods inside.

To make matters worse, your DNA can play a role in how well you naturally detox. See, most of us can handle the toxins we come across in our daily lives (if we're not overstressed and if there aren't too many of them). But with a slight genetic differ-ence here or there, that ability might not exist in you. Or it might be hampered by something that happened in your child-hood, when you were in utero, or even two generations before you were born. *That* kind of hampering, along with the role of DNA, is discussed in Chapter 6.

But we promise there *is good news in this book*! And it begins in Chapter 7, where you can learn how to find out if you have a toxic body burden. Then Chapter 8 follows up with information on how detoxification works.

Of course, once you get clean, you want to stay clean. But we do live in a dirty world. So Chapters 9 and 10 will help you battle the toxins that are always trying to invade your body.

Because detoxification is just one part of your health, we end the book by discussing the five core areas to focus on in order to live a healthy, vital, and long life. It is through that lens that Ed and I treat our patients so that they can go from just living to actually thriving.

We're Supposed to Get Better with Age

At Five Journeys, we reject the notion that you are meant to get a chronic illness and die without full mental capacity sometime in your seventies. We believe that the body wants to be well. When we provide what it lacks and remove what is a burden, the body will heal itself. By detoxing, you remove those burdens.

That philosophy has been at the core of our practice since 2008. We don't treat a symptom to make it go away or hide. We treat the body as a whole, so it can heal itself. That's what Functional Medicine is all about.

I think Ed always knew he wanted to be in Functional Medicine. Me? I never knew there was an option other than conventional medicine! I went to medical school without any real thought about what I would do after graduation. I attended a rigorous, year-round program that took all the tenacity I could muster. It was a dual program, at the end of which I received my MBA in healthcare administration as well as an MD and went on to become an OB/GYN.

Although thinking I would become a conventional doctor, I had always been a bit of a maverick in my education. I never settled for the standard answers. More than once, I (unintentionally) annoyed my professors by asking why questions about what was happening. Like, "Why don't we give a prescription for probiotics along with the Diflucan to balance their poor vaginas?" Subsequently, I wasn't very popular with them. But I didn't care. I wanted to know how best to treat my future patients.

Meanwhile, Ed, who had never accepted that there is only one right answer to anything, had become immersed in studying a broad range of treatment modalities between college and medical school. By the time he was admitted into the MD/PhD program at Boston University, he had studied shiatsu, Japanese bodywork, acupuncture, energy medicine, and more, while also doing basic research at the Dana-Farber Cancer Center.

After graduation, Ed was mentored in Functional Medicine, which focuses on the whole patient, not just the patient's symptoms. Ed's mentor diagnosed me with celiac disease, something I felt should have been discovered years, if not a couple of decades, earlier. And that's when I realized I wanted to be on their team too. I wanted to practice Functional Medicine; it had provided the answer I needed, and I wanted to do the same for my patients.

So Ed and I started our first practice, which became the largest Functional Medicine practice in the nation during its time. Eight years later, we launched our membership-based wellness organization, Five Journeys, where we continue to help patients achieve extraordinary health results.

But a practice and an education do not necessarily mean a doctor has all the answers. And, really, no one has all the answers for everyone. What we do, however, is take a systematic approach to health, wellness, and healing that tends to improve many illnesses. We believe that each disease has its basis in imbalance and inflammation. So we get cracking on figuring out the root cause of those. We have helped, and continue to help, thousands of patients with our approach. On top of that, I practice what I preach. I'm living the treatments, and I'm doing what I tell my patients to do.

I've spent the past fourteen years h*ll-bent on walking the path of good health. My toxic profile and detox protocols are just part of that journey. Not only will I continue this journey for the rest of my life, but I'm putting it in this book in the hopes that you will use it as a template to help you get better too. I did the heavy lifting already, so you have a roadmap to help you heal and spend the least amount of time possible suffering from toxicity.

We believe you are supposed to get better with age. Unfortunately, for many of us, toxins build up in our bodies over time and don't cause problems until we are older, which makes it hard to be vintage and vital. But remember, there's good news here! Detox isn't age-dependent. We can help our bodies detox and heal at any age. We can live as happy and healthy in our eighties as we did in our twenties—even happier and healthier!

Let's Get Cleaning

As you progress through this book, it might feel a bit over-whelming to discover there is so much to think about and do. Seriously, I know—been there, *still* doing that. Completely cleaning your life to have a body as toxin-free as possible will be an ongoing process. Understand this, though: you will never be completely toxin-free. But you *can* get the major toxins down and keep them at a low enough level that your body can handle them and not let them build up and make you sick. Yes, that requires an entire overhaul of everything you do. However, just as with Rome, it doesn't need to be done in one day.

If you feel discouraged by how much is involved in detoxification and living a clean life, just pick one place to start. And then, when you master that, pick another, then another, and iteratively build on your successes. At the end of each chapter, we'll list our Hot Top Tips of clean behavior that will be a good starting point for you, even if it's just something little. Remember, little things add up to big things!

And know that you don't have to do it alone. You can get help (as you'll see in Chapter 8). And maybe you should. The last thing detoxification should be is stressful! As you'll soon see, stress only makes toxicity worse. But first, let's talk about why we're so toxic to begin with.

CHAPTER 1

Dirty Girls
Go Bald

I'll never forget the day my hairstylist acknowledged my truth. I'd spent months trying to force her to do it, but Patty wouldn't budge. She always told me I was beautiful, that my hair was gorgeous, and that nothing was wrong.

I wanted to believe her. But I suspected she was trying to avoid what was so clear to me. Maybe she just couldn't bring herself to risk hurting my feelings by telling me the truth. Maybe she thought it would piss me off if she told me what she knew I *really* didn't want to hear despite my repeated imploring. Regardless, at every appointment for many months, I would ask, "Patty, do you think I'm losing my hair?" And she would always assure me I wasn't. She'd insist my hair looked just like it always had.

But I knew it didn't. And eventually she had to admit the truth. "Well, actually, now that you mention it, yes," she finally said after I'd shoved the back of my head into her face once again. "I don't know what's going on. But yeah. You're losing your hair."

She could have stopped there, but she didn't. "Pretty rapidly too," she added.

There were so many things wrong with that moment, I was tempted to crumple on the floor and cry. But I didn't. Someone else's hair was all over it. Instead, I did what every other rational and intelligent woman would do. I went home and vowed to get to the bottom of whatever was taking my hair away.

Ugh. I felt like the universe was against me. I didn't deserve this. I did everything a healthy woman was supposed to do. And I didn't have any vices (if you exclude my regular overuse of the F-word). Granted, I probably didn't get as much sleep as I needed, but that's because I'm a mom. I wasn't a "bad mom" out carousing around at clubs all night. Moms just don't get the kind of sleep they need, and yet not all of us were losing our hair. Why was I?

The day Patty admitted the truth to me was in December. It then took a few months for me to think it through, to figure it out, and to recognize that what was going on with my body was not normal. So life went on like normal for a while. I worked. I took care of my family. I even went on vacation. My hair loss accelerated after our vacation, so I finally got my act together to do mold and heavy metals testing. Fast-forward six months and I'm on a detox protocol to remove mycotoxins and heavy metals from my body, and guess what? My hair had stopped falling out.

That was great news: I'd found the problem. It turns out that my body was storing toxins, including lead and mercury, and I had been losing hair because of it. Actually, I had been suffering an annoying number of symptoms for years because of it; I just never knew what was going on. I mean, why would I be so toxic? Remember, I was the poster child for clean living! How did I get so polluted? So dirty? It's not like I ate melted plastic as a child or played with liquid mercury or...oh, wait a minute.

Actually, I had.

Before you start thinking I was some kind of a misfit child with peculiar habits, let me assure you I had a typical, normal upbringing. Probably very similar to yours. Which is why it's important that you hear my story before your hair starts falling out too.

We're Born behind the Eight Ball

I was born into a middle-class family that lived in a middle-class neighborhood in Massachusetts. My toxic exposure, though, began before I was born. When you look at my genetic profile, you can see I should have been put into a bubble and protected from life as soon as I exited my mother's womb. Instead, I had the next best thing: my mother breastfed me. Yes, it's one of the best things you can do for your baby as far as nourishment goes. But, unfortunately, my mother had been exposed to quite a bit of common pollutants in the 1960s and heavy metals throughout her whole life. Things like polychlorinated biphenyls (PCBs) had filled the air she breathed and contaminated her body. Then, when she had me, she unknowingly shared that toxicity with me in some beautiful moments of maternal love and care. You see, one of the ways a female body detoxifies is through breast milk.

Yes, we still believe breast milk is the best thing you can feed your baby. If you're already doing it, keep doing it. If you're currently pregnant, breastfeed your baby! But if you are not pregnant and are thinking about having a baby in the future, it might be a good thing to do some testing and see if you should detox first. Detoxification should never happen when you're pregnant or nursing, though.

As a baby and toddler, I did what nature programmed me to do: put my hands in my mouth. That in and of itself is a normal thing. However, the home I grew up in was built in an era when lead paint was also a normal thing. One of the most common ways for children to be exposed to lead is via common household dust. Don't get me wrong; my mother kept a clean house! But our home did what every building does: it expanded and contracted with temperature changes and, as it did so, microscopic lead particles would slough off. So it's very easy to see how my slobbery hands would pick up those lead particles and place them directly where my toddler mind thought everything should go: in my mouth.

Eventually, when I was able to walk on two feet on a regular basis, I learned the joy of sloppy joes—made with ground meat and a powdered flavoring and served on a glutinous bun, just what a celiac-waiting-to-happen doesn't need. My family also indulged in most of the convenient, easy-to-prepare foods that came out of boxes and pouches. Everybody did back then—and still does! Mac and cheese, Hamburger Helper, and many others—they were everywhere because they were so convenient. Usually, all you had to do was mix some water into the chemicals in the package, add that to some pasta, rice, or a casserole, and voilà! Delicious meals filled with all sorts of artificial ingredients.

Soon, as with most of my peers, I got to experience the dentist's chair. I was there more than once to get a filling for a cavity. And back then the most common ingredient for those fillings was mercury-containing amalgam.

Oh, but then came the microwave in the 1980s. Who knew what a joy bombarding food with plastic particles could be? We microwaved everything, including all the newly introduced foods that came in plastic! Again, it was normal. It was convenient. Frankly, the microwave was considered a modern miracle. Unfortunately, maybe we overreacted with that "miracle" label because, as it turns out, when you heat food in plastic, the chemicals from the plastic leach into your food and become part of your meal. And they're not friendly chemicals! As you'll see in Chapter 4, plastics can be very bad for your health.

I could go on and on discussing all the toxins I was exposed to in my youth, but you probably have a good idea by now. I'm sure many other women my age had similar exposures and similar upbringings. Though I do wonder if I'm the only one who ever played with balls of mercury in high school when a thermometer broke.

> **Do you know what your microwave is good for? Killing plants.**
>
> **Our daughter did a science experiment in which she had two identical plants kept in the same area. One of them she watered with water she had heated up on a Bunsen burner and then let cool before applying to the plant.**
>
> **The other plant she watered with water she heated in a microwave and then let cool.**
>
> **The Bunsen burner plant thrived. The microwave plant died.**

Now, do you really think it's a good idea to eat or drink anything that has been heated in a microwave? We "divorced" our microwave after that little experiment!

Is Everyone in Danger?

You might be thinking my situation is an extreme one. I mean, I live in the Northeast, the part of the country that invented acid rain. Why should anyone be surprised that I wound up loaded with toxins?

But let me assure you—well, maybe assure isn't the right word—let me caution you: if you're alive in the twenty-first century, you've probably had too much exposure to too many toxins. But if most of your life was lived in the twentieth century, don't think you're protected; the twentieth century was just as dirty.

We started really polluting our Earth, and hence our bodies, back in the industrial revolution when we discovered we could burn fossil fuels. That's when, simultaneously, we invented black smoke and suddenly charcoal gray was the color of the year every year for fashionistas. It was hard to keep your bright pinks vibrant and pretty with all that soot in the air.

Since then, humanity has been h*ll-bent on inventing as many new-to-nature molecules as possible, and many of them are based on petroleum, which is just toxic for us to ingest, absorb, inhale, or any other in- you can think of.[1] While creating those inventions, we poisoned our waters, our air, and the soil we grow our foods in, and so far humans have proven themselves to be kinds of beings who clean as they go. We wait until rivers catch on fire before we think we should clean them up, and, meanwhile, our oceans have layers of plastic lining the floors and permeating the fat of the fish we eat. Instead of reducing the carbon overload in the air, we chop down the trees that replenish our oxygen and use them for fire, which then adds more carbon. Then that poisoned water and toxic air are filtered through our soils, making it contaminated before we plant our genetically modified and pesticide-sprayed seeds.

Granted, now that we are postindustrial, most governments around the world have put some limits on what corporations can spew into our air and water—but those are limits per day, and they vary by city, state, and country. They're still spewing, so ultimately there is a cumulative effect in the air and water.

---

1 New York State Attorney General, "What Are the Health Effects of Exposure to Petroleum Products?" https://ag.ny.gov/environmental/oil-spill/what-are-health-effects-exposure-petroleum-products.

These industrial toxicants get into your food via leaching into the groundwater that is then used to irrigate commercial crops. It is sprayed directly onto and absorbed by the crops that you eat or that are fed to the animals you subsequently eat. Things like insect repellents, herbicides, and fungicides don't just protect the crops; they *infect* them, which means they infect *you* with those chemicals. And some of them are really bad actors.

Toxicant or Toxin? What's the Difference?

The difference between these two words is found in their origins. A toxicant is used to refer to man-made toxic substances, like industrial by-products. A toxin, on the other hand, is something that is produced naturally, like the stuff that oozes out of the skin of those poison dart frogs in South America.

Another bad actor is plastic! Everything, it seems, has some form of plastic in it, which means—because plastic isn't good about keeping to itself—everything has plastic particles inside it. Our oceans are so full of plastic that the fish we eat actually have plastic particles in them. It's estimated that up to 36 percent of wild fish have plastics in them (and, in some accounts, 100 percent of filter fish like mussels, clams, and oysters).[2] And yes, we're eating that plastic, too, when we eat fish.

Plastic is made, in part, from diethyl phthalate. That's a chemical that is used to make plastics more flexible. It is used in packaging, toys, automobile parts, and more. Sure, it's useful to have flexible plastic, but particles of it get released into the air from the factories, and then we breathe it in, we absorb it into our skin, and when it contaminates our groundwater, we're at risk of drinking it or eating foods grown with that water. In addition to that, when it's in food packaging, we're at risk of it melting into our foods before we eat them.

What's so bad about diethyl phthalate? Well, they put you at risk for problems like impeded blood coagulation, low testosterone, autoimmune disease, altered sexual development in children, reproductive damage, and depressive leukocyte function. According to one researcher, they are responsible for increasing rates of infertility and "cause sperm cells to basically commit suicide."[3] Oh, and they cause cancer.

---

2 The Conversation, "Hundreds of Fish Species, Including Many That Humans Eat, Are Consuming Plastic," *EcoWatch*, February 14, 2021, www.ecowatch. com/fish-consuming-plastic-2650530342.html#:~:text=Our%20research%20 revealed%20that%20marine,those%20species%20had%20ingested%20plas- tic.;%20www.blastic.eu/knowledge-bank/impacts/plastic-ngestion/fish/#:~:tex- t=The%20percentage%20of%20fish%20that,plastic%20from%20the%20gastro- intestinal%20tract.

3 Bijal P. Trivedi, "The Everyday Chemicals That Might Be Leading Us to Our Ex- tinction," *New York Times*, March 5, 2021, www.nytimes.com/2021/03/05/books/ review/shanna-swan-count-down.html?referringSource=articleShare.

In the chorus of their song "Dirty Water," released in 1965, the band the Standells sang about the polluted Charles River in Massachusetts, where there were large fish kills, plumes of chemical smoke arising from the surface, and pollutants so thick they would turn the water pink and orange. Since then, there have been strenuous efforts to clean the river up, but the work is ongoing. The toxic sediment on the bottom is so dangerous that swimmers can only jump in the deeper parts from a dock so they cannot touch bottom, and if anyone is found swimming without a permit, they are fined $250.

As with plastics and diethyl phthalates, many of the pollutants damaging our bodies are really leftovers from things that we love and need—like mechanisms that have been invented over the last couple of centuries for our convenience or safety (how ironic, eh?) Lead pipes are a good example.

Yes, many of us still have lead pipes bringing water into our homes and workspaces. Easily available, clean running water, I think we all can agree, is a wonderful thing. Lead? Not so much. And if your pipes are lead-free, your fixtures may not be. Also, lead's floating in the air around us from buildings getting torn down, being improperly renovated, or just existing. Any structure built before 1978 is at risk for having lead in the paint. For those buildings, even if they've been repainted, as time wears away at them, dust is created that gets blown around, falls on the ground, and is picked up on the bottom of shoes and brought to wherever you live. Lead happens!

You wanna know how tricky lead is? Ed and I have seen numerous female patients over the years who were diagnosed with osteoporosis or osteopenia. They've been told it's because they are menopausal and, well, that just happens sometimes, and perhaps they should have drunk more milk when they were younger.

But that's not the truth. The truth is, as our testing proves, these women are often loaded with lead! The body doesn't store all its toxins in fat; some go right to our bones. And when lead heads there, it prevents calcium from entering. Those women could drink milk until the cows come home (pun intended) and never get strong bones—until they get the lead out!

Pollutants that were invented to help us stay safe are found in items like flame retardants, which are applied to most mattresses as well as to other soft furnishings and some of your clothing (in fact, probably all of your children's pajamas and Halloween costumes have flame retardants on them). Sure, it sounds like a good idea to have a mattress that won't go up in flames when you're sleeping on it. But think it through. Why were flame retardants put on mattresses to begin with? Because, back in the day, in overcrowded places like tenement buildings, someone would fall asleep while smoking in bed. Their mattress would catch on fire and then burn down the entire building, possibly the entire city block.

How many of us live in overcrowded tenement buildings now? How many of us smoke in bed? Okay...if you're smoking in bed, then you *should* probably sleep on a mattress with flame retardants. But if you're not, then maybe you shouldn't risk poisoning yourself with the off-gassing chemicals from your mattress.

So, as you can see, exposure to toxins is something that's almost impossible to avoid. I mean, even if you sold everything you owned and lived aboard a sailboat in the middle of the ocean, you'd still have to contend with eating toxic fish for dinner.

That's It! I Can't Take Any More!

My body did its best to handle the onslaught of toxins I'd been exposed to. But it had reached its saturation point about a year before I confronted Patty. I'm pretty sure the tipping point for my body happened the day I heard some loud noises outside my house. I looked through an open window and realized my neighbor was knocking down his 1940s postwar house. The air grew heavy with the dirt and crap floating around from it. I kind of panicked and forced everyone to shut all the windows because I was afraid there might be lead particles in the vicinity.

I was probably right, but I didn't think much about it after we shut the windows. Then, nine months later, Ed and I went to

Paris on vacation. It was shortly after the Notre Dame fire. I remember remarking to him that it was very dusty in Paris that spring.

I was definitely right that time. The dust was heavy because it was filled with ash and other particles from the fire.[4] Particles that were loaded with lead from the multiple layers of paint that had once covered the surfaces inside the cathedral. Particles that we breathed in the whole time we were there. Particles we absorbed into our skin as we held hands walking down the Champs-Élysées. Particles that we unintentionally ate because they landed on our food as we dined at outdoor cafés.

When we came back to the States, my body just couldn't take any more toxicity. You see, the body is resilient until it hits a certain point, and then something has to give. In my case, my somethings included clear thinking, as my brain became increasingly foggy; my waistline, as a layer of unmeltable fat clung to me; and my hair. My hair, which was the straw that broke the camel's back.

So you can be someone doing all the right things, you can be like me and join me on that poster for clean living, and *still* be unable to protect yourself from all the toxins on the planet today. But, as I promised in the introduction, there is good news. If you suspect you might be a dirty girl (or boy), there are plenty of things you can do to clean up your act. It's a matter of taking an inventory of your life to see from where the potential toxins are coming to you, finding out if you are, indeed, toxic,

---

4 Elian Peltier et al., "Notre-Dame's Toxic Fallout," New York Times, September 14, 2019, www.nytimes.com/interactive/2019/09/14/world/europe/notre-dame-fire-lead.html.

and then getting some help to detox. However, there is something we need to talk about first.

That something is stress. It might sound crazy, but stress can be the deciding factor that determines whether you become a hot toxic mess in the first place. And should you become one, stress can hinder your ability to detox. So let's see how stress works in our bodies, so that we can get it to work *for* us, not against us.

Hot Top Tips

1. Stop using your microwave, and definitely don't nuke plastic!

2. Consider safely replacing your mercury-filled amalgam fillings with composites. (Consult your dentist— better yet, find a biological dentist to help!)

3. Ditch plastic food-storage containers.

4. Evaluate your house for lead—do you know when it was built? When was the plumbing put in?

5. Search the web for easy-to-prepare meals. You'll discover there are ways to make meals from fresh vegetables and ingredients that are just as quick and easy as anything from a box.

CHAPTER 2

Sex or Stress

To get an understanding of how stress impacts your body, let's take a look at what I call the Holy Trinity of Stress Organs: the liver, adrenals, and gut. Sure, you're living in the twenty-first century where the odds of being eaten alive by a saber-toothed tiger are relatively slim. However, your body's stress response hasn't caught up with your modern-day lifestyle. It still views your life through a very primitive lens. What that means is, when your boss yells at you, or when you get a call from your child's teacher, or when you watch the news on TV, your body responds as if it's about to be attacked by that tiger. To protect your life, the Holy Trinity of Stress Organs kicks in the fight-flight-or-freeze response.

Your liver stops focusing on toxin removal and releases stored glucose into your bloodstream so that you have energy to escape the wild animal that your body thinks is chasing you. After all, that tiger is about to eat you! You need to run and run fast. To do that, your muscles need fuel. And sugar is a great fuel. So the liver yells, "Stop the presses!" and shuts its detox factory down in order to churn out sugar in the form of glucose. Once the sugar gets going to fuel your run, the liver will start producing cholesterol as a backup fuel. How surprising is that? Your liver creates the things that make you fat or prone to a heart attack in response to stress.

That sugar and cholesterol could be very beneficial. If you do happen to need to climb a mountain to get away from the tiger, they will make your success possible. Ever hear the urban legend about an eighty-pound woman lifting a car off her baby? I've often wondered how her baby got under the car to begin with, but I've never questioned the superhuman ability that stress can create. Unfortunately, if you're not running away from that tiger in real life, or lifting a car off your baby, and instead are in a meeting, chewing on the inside of your cheek while your a**hole boss blames your team for something you didn't do, then instead of using up all that energy to escape, your body stores it in fat. New fat. Fat that usually finds a home around your midsection, you know, in the muffin-top area.

Meanwhile, in conjunction with the liver's efforts to save you, the adrenals turn on their cortisol factory and pump that hormone into your bloodstream. Cortisol does a number of things in your body, most of which involve your energy levels. During times of stress, it focuses on getting that glucose rushing through your system and on shutting down what it deems nonessential-for-the-moment bodily functions. See, it's seldom a good time to make a pit stop to poop when you're running for your life. So cortisol shuts down your digestive system, and then the energy that would be required to digest food is diverted to your legs, so you can run. It has a similar effect on the immune system, the reproductive system, and the growth process. All that stuff gets shut down until the immediate threat to your endangered life has passed.

So while the liver and adrenals are focused on getting you the h*ll out of Dodge, the gut is feeling like an ignored step-child. Without the liver and pancreas providing the required resources to break down food in the belly, and because cortisol has shut down any hope of emptying whatever is there anyway, the gut is stuck with food rotting in it.

Sometimes it's unfortunate that we're *not* being chased by prehistoric predators—our modern stress doesn't always have a neat and tidy end. We don't make it to the cave where the roaring fire scares away the beasts as we relax and draw pictures on the wall. Instead, we leave our nasty boss to fight traffic all the way home, where we deal with the angry teacher call, worry about our parents' health and our children's futures, and fear the stock market and worldwide calamities that the news media keep showing us. All the while, we're juggling the car pool, making dinner, finding last-minute supplies for science fairs, doing yet another load of never-ending laundry, and *Ugh! Who thought it would be a good idea to make the dog a collar out of chewing gum?!*

So, for us, in our busy lives, our stress sometimes doesn't seem to end—it's chronic. And now, because we're *not* burning off all that new sugar and cholesterol in flight, the fat grows and the body processes remain slow or even stop. To make matters worse, when stress is prolonged, the liver just doesn't have the resources left to deal with the toxins that are coming into our bodies. And remember the gut's situation? All that rotting food wreaks havoc on our digestive system: nutrient absorption is impaired, bad bacteria thrives in our intestines, and gas is produced.

But it gets worse! When you're under stress, something called methylation is one of the processes your body shuts down to give you energy. Methylation is part of your body's natural detoxification strategy.

See, the way your body naturally detoxes stuff is by making it easier to eliminate. And yes, by eliminate, I mean pee, poop, or sweat, which requires toxins to be water-soluble. Unfortunately, most toxins and hormones are fat-soluble. When your body is fully functioning, not overburdened, and not over stressed, your liver has the ability to attach a methyl group (this is a fancy term for one carbon molecule that's connected to three hydrogen molecules) to your toxins and hormones, which makes them water-soluble. You then dump those methylated items into your urine or stool, or you sweat them out.

In short, all that stress makes us fat, bloated, and toxic.

Not Tonight, Honey. I've Got Cortisol

Cortisol is not necessarily a bad thing. In fact, you do need it in your body. Without it, you die. However, for optimum health, your cortisol can't be too high (or too low). Unrelieved stress can make it go high and stay high. When you're thinking about the things you need to order, the appointments you need to schedule, the interactions you had with your neighbor about fixing the fence, and so on, you're jacking up your cortisol by stressing yourself out. And that has nothing to do with the external factors, like a global pandemic or recession, election year, and so on, constantly boosting the cortisol output.

The thing is, your body is programmed to thrive when things are balanced. When one hormone is off, then many others get thrown off. And cortisol is no exception. When it remains elevated, it can unbalance many of your other hormones, including your sex hormones, which will tank your sex drive.

Seriously, especially for women in menopause, you *cannot* produce cortisol at the same time as you produce your sex hormones. As women enter menopause, the ovaries hand over the responsibility of making sex hormones (estrogen, testosterone, and progesterone) to the adrenals. When your adrenals are in fight-flight-or-freeze mode, they don't have capacity to make cortisol *and* fuel your sex drive. That's why when you're a stress ball, the last thing you want is for the hubs to wink at you over the dinner table.

The imbalance of those sex hormones coming from your adrenals also fuels your hot flashes and night sweats—everybody says "my hormones are off," and they think it's normal menopause. It's not. It's stress!

The same can be said about cortisol for men (granted, not the menopause part). For men, the big worry is cortisol "steal." See, cortisol uses the same pathways in your body as testosterone, and there's only room for one hormone in that pathway! So if men are making too much cortisol, they are decreasing their testosterone production. In other words, either you're stressing out and pushing cortisol through your body or you're chilling and letting the testosterone come out to play.

Sex or stress? It's your choice!

It's a Balancing Act

Because there will never be a time in your life when you do not have some kind of stress, one of the most important things you can do for your health is to figure out how to manage it so that you can support methylation and naturally detox (and get extra friendly with your mate again).

When it comes to stress symptoms and other physical complaints, we like to use the analogy of a rain barrel. A rain barrel fills up a little at a time. At some point, there's an overflow valve to let the excess water escape to an appropriate outlet, but if it's plugged due to a lack of maintenance, the water will fill up the barrel and then overflow. Similarly, if you don't give your stress a chance to dissipate, it will overflow into your life.

When we reach that overflow point, the combination of prolonged or sustained stress and a growing exposure to an onslaught of toxins will cause our bodies to stop focusing on even *trying* to detox. Instead, your body will start storing the toxins in fat cells, bones, and tissue, while hoping and praying that one day you will have the time to deal with them. But if the toxins keep coming and the stress doesn't ease up, something else has to give. Rain barrels will leak and burst. Your body can develop symptoms like insomnia, skin rashes (eczema, psoriasis), high blood pressure, aching joints, allergies, anxiety, depression, irritable bowel, weight loss or gain, hair loss, and the list goes on and on.

Every person's body is different, so the overflow point is also different for everyone. Often, there's something major that really sets things off: a car accident, a traumatic breakup, being out of your home country for an extended period of time, a virus, taking care of a very sick family member, or something else. But sometimes there isn't one clear moment. Instead, you just slide into a chronic state of not feeling well.

What I find interesting is that everyone admits they're stressed. They just seem to take it for granted that life is stressful and that's normal. But I don't think many people realize just *how* stressed—that is, overstressed—they are. So here's a questionnaire called the Perceived Stress Scale (PSS) from Mind Garden (www.mindgarden.com) to help you gauge the level of stress you've had to deal with that may be impacting your life.[5]

For each question, think about your feelings and thoughts over the last month only. Then, for each, assign a level number that most corresponds to you.

Level 0 = Never

Level 1 = Almost Never

Level 2 = Sometimes

Level 3 = Fairly Often

Level 4 = Very Often

---

5 Reprinted with permission from Sheldon Cohen, Tom Kamarck, and Robin Mermelstein, "A Global Measure of Perceived Stress," *Journal of Health and Social Behavior* 24, no. 4 (1983): 385–396.

	QUESTION	LEVEL	SCORE
1	In the last month, how often have you been upset because of something that happened unexpectedly?		
2	In the last month, how often have you felt that you were unable to control the important things in your life?		
3	In the last month, how often have you felt nervous and "stressed"?		
4	In the last month, how often have you felt confident about your ability to handle your personal problems?		
5	In the last month, how often have you felt that things were going your way?		
6	In the last month, how often have you found that you could not cope with all the things that you had to do?		
7	In the last month, how often have you been able to control irritations in your life?		
8	In the last month, how often have you felt that you were on top of things?		
9	In the last month, how often have you been angered because of things that were outside of your control?		
10	In the last month, how often have you felt difficulties were piling up so high that you could not overcome them?		

Now you can calculate your total PSS score.

- For your answers in 4, 5, 7, and 8, enter the following scores based on your number:

    * Level 0 = Score of 4

    * Level 1 = Score of 3

    * Level 2 = Score of 2

    * Level 3 = Score of 1

    * Level 4 = Score of 0

- For your answers in 1, 2, 3, 6, 9, and 10, your score will equal your level answer. So for those:

    * Level 0 = Score of 0

    * Level 1 = Score of 1

    * Level 2 = Score of 2

    * Level 3 = Score of 3

    * Level 4 = Score of 4

- Now add up all your scores.

- Scores can range from 0 (which is laughable, right? We *all* have some stress in our lives) to 40. It's generally accepted that:[6]

    * Scores from 0 to 13 are seen as indicating low stress.

    * Scores between 14 and 26 are considered moderate stress levels.

    * Scores over 27 suggest high perceived stress.

Now that you've read through *why* stress is not the best thing for your health, you know that if you're on the higher end of this scale, then you need to find a way to deal with your stress. We suggest you pick your top three stressors and create a plan for how you are going to deal with them. You have a choice with everything. If your job is a top stressor, you can change your job *or* you can change your relationship with it. The same can be said for a marriage or partnership, for a family situation, for anything.

As with any change, it takes more than just the commitment. You'll need a plan and a date to revisit it every week, or month, or however frequently is good for you to check on your progress or decide if you need help. Because, regardless of how you got there, you have to find a way to deal with your stress, or no effort of detoxing will give you the good health results you are looking for.

We could write an entire separate book—h*ll, we could write a series of books—about how to manage stress. Though that's not the point of this book, we do want to give you a direction in which to go. So here are some of the top methods for easing stress that many of our clients have found success with:

- Regular exercise, particularly yoga

- Talk therapy

- Setting yourself up for a good night's sleep, maybe some soothing herbal tea or a relaxing bath before bed. Eliminating your exposure to blue light from electronic devices. Writing in a gratitude journal for a few minutes before tucking in for the night.

- Meditation. There is a related practice called "forest bathing" that Dr. Qing Li describes in his book Forest Bathing: How Trees Can Help You Find Health and Happiness. Basically, you choose a natural place or forest where it would be safe for you to walk—leaving your phone behind you or on do-not-disturb. Enter the forest and walk aimlessly, slowly; with no intention of getting to someplace in particular, let your body be your guide. Be mindful and aware of the sights, sound, smells, and everything you can experience. Let nature and the forest be a peaceful sanctuary for you.

- Ask for help! Many of us just don't think to ask our part-
  ners, friends, or family for help. Get the kids involved,
  even. None of us should own a superhero cape! We need
  to stop expecting ourselves to do it all and to set boundaries for what we can realistically do. That means no
  more overcommitting and learning to say *no*.

- Laugh. Finding something so humorous that you get a
  good belly laugh actually improves your circulation and
  helps your muscles relax, both of which are excellent
  de-stressors.[7]

- Be kind to yourself. While the old Stuart Smalley skits
  might provide some laughter, the idea behind his prac-
  tices can actually be a stress-reliever. Repeating positive
  affirmations to give yourself encouragement, to treat
  yourself with compassion, and to speak with uncondi-
  tional acceptance and love to yourself attenuates stress.[8]

The above ideas are just a few to get you started. Choose any
of them as a starting point to ameliorate your stress level now.
Then make a plan to tackle the actual stressors in your life.

Granted, we know if stress were easy to deal with, none of us
would be stressed out. But a really cool thing is that the behav-

7 Mayo Clinic Staff, "Stress Relief from Laughter? It's No Joke," Mayo Founda-
tion for Medical Education and Research, April 5, 2019, www.mayoclinic.org/
healthy-lifestyle/stress-management/in-depth/stress-relief/art-20044456.

8 David K. Sherman et al., "Psychological Vulnerability and Stress: The Effects of
Self-Affirmation on Sympathetic Nervous System Responses to Naturalistic Stressors," *Health Psychology* 28, no. 5 (2009): 554–562., doi:10.1037/a0014663.

iors you need to change in order to clean up your life—eating better foods, getting better sleep, creating a healthier environment—will all help your body manage stress better. However, if you can eliminate one particular toxin, you will achieve the biggest reduction in your stress levels. And that poison is toxic relationships.

Cleaning Up Toxic Relationships

Toxic relationships are so stressful that they are just as bad for our health as environmental toxins. When I see patients in toxic relationships, I counsel them to make sure they understand that even though we have supercool tools, treatments, and interventions, most of them will be useless until they deal with their single most detrimental health issue. Every once in a while, we'll see someone who really does need to get out of a bad marriage or leave a bad job before they can heal their bodies. Unfortunately, even the greatest supplements in the world are useless against the toxicity of extremely unhealthy social constructs. The pain for people in situations like that is all-encompassing and is just too big to walk around; it's like a giant boulder in the middle of the road. We can't work around it to heal their body. They have to remove it first.

Unfortunately, toxic relationships come in all shapes and sizes. Some we're born into. Some are in the friend and social groups we're affiliated with. Some are with our own habits—meaning those of us who *must* constantly watch the news or follow negative feeds on social media are in toxic relationships with our habits. And some of us are in toxic relationships with ourselves; we're the ones who engage in negative self-talk, take on responsibilities we shouldn't, and beat ourselves up for minor mistakes while never celebrating our accomplishments.

Listen, our brains are supercomputers. Everything that gets programmed into them controls how they work. So if you're consistently putting in negative input—whether it's from negative people in your life, social media, the news, yourself, whatever—that's going to impact you in the form of stress and negative output. You need to detox from all those toxic relationships.

Now I know that it's not always possible to cut people out of your life. But if you want to get better physically, eliminating, or at least reducing the exposure to, toxic relationships is necessary. If you're in a soul-sapping job, even if it pays well, and you know you should be doing something else, *that* depletes your energy. Through changes in diet, lifestyle, and the addition of high-quality supplements, we might be able to get you to feel physically better by 20 percent, but the job is draining you every day. There's only so much we'll be able to do for you.

And realize that it's not the fault of the job. The job might be completely fine. It's the relationship between you and the job that is (sometimes literally) killing you. Meanwhile, there are other jobs out there. So you'll need to find something else to truly get better.

Similarly, you might be in a relationship with a great person— who just isn't the right one for you. So if you are committed to being healthy, you have to detox from your relationship with your partner.

Now What?

By now you should have an idea of how stress could be impacting your life. If it's barely a blip on your life radar, then congratulations! You're managing stress well, and the rest of the book will just be sugar-free icing on the gluten-free cake.

If, however, it's a big deal in your life, the remaining chapters may seem overwhelming, at first. It can be a lot to take in, so take it a chapter at a time. Read what you can handle, then when you're ready, come back to the book and read some more.

And now that you have an understanding of how stress is a toxin and how it can impact your health, let's move on to talk about the toxins in foods because that might be the easiest (hence least stressful) place for you to make changes.

Hot Top Tips

1. Take a three-day social media and/or news detox.

2. Get off the grid for a day (or a week if you can swing it!). Yes, it's a major change to go without news, internet connection, or alerts on your phone, but it's something that can have a truly beneficial effect on your well-being.

3. Inventory your relationships. Are any toxic? If so, start working on a plan to distance or divest.

4. Identify one thing you can do daily to de-stress—then do it. Remember, meditation doesn't require a membership, transportation, or anything other than a few minutes of your focus. Consider taking up a meditation practice. You can, if you think it would be helpful, find a teacher or use one of the many apps available for your smartphone. You'd be surprised what wonders ten to twenty minutes of meditation in the morning can do for you.

5. Catch yourself in the middle of negative self-talk and change the script. Instead of "I'm so bad at this," say "I haven't mastered this *yet*, but I'm working on it!"

CHAPTER 3

Eat, Drink, and Be Toxic

By the time Emily made it to us, she was sick as sh*t! At just over thirty years old, this once vibrant, energetic, and brilliant young woman sitting in our office was a shell of a human being.

The medical history provided by her primary care doctor said her symptoms began about three years prior. What started out as headaches and the desire for a nap in the afternoon had grown to the need to sleep more hours of the day than she was awake. And now it didn't make much difference whether Emily was horizontal and conked out or upright with eyes wide open: she had very little motivation to do *any*thing and was emotionally distant.

It was explained to us that she and her husband worked for a startup that had hit the ground running. On top of being crazy busy getting their company cranking, they had purchased their first home, which piled on to her responsibilities. So when the desire for a nap originally hit in the afternoons, it seemed natural. Who wouldn't be tired with all Emily had going on? Knowing she was overextended energy-wise, she indulged the naps. But then their lengths grew—even after she started going to bed earlier and waking up later—and yet she never felt she was getting enough sleep.

Soon, it became apparent that her memory was slipping. And as lethargy replaced her alertness, she lost the ability to think clearly. She also lost the ability to do math, which for some of us might not seem all that important, but not only was she typically good at math, she needed it for her business! She *needed* to function in general and just couldn't.

Eventually, the perpetual state of brain fog became so dense that no lighthouse on the Eastern Seaboard could penetrate it. She needed help!

Since she was referred to us from her primary care doctor, we knew she'd had the basic blood work and testing done, so we skipped ahead and ran a series of toxicology tests. Sure enough, her body was loaded with lead. In fact, she had the highest level of lead toxicity we had ever seen. Her husband had a high level too, which helped us figure out the source. It had to be from a place they both frequented and someplace new to them when the symptoms began. In other words, it had to be from their new-to-them home, which was old enough to have lead pipes in the plumbing.

When we do heavy metals testing (lead and mercury, for example), we like to see levels under eight. Anything over eight gets our attention. Sixteen or above is considered significant. Sometimes, we get people (particularly older people who have been exposed for longer periods of time) who are in the thirty-to-fifty range, occasionally as high as between seventy and eighty. However, this patient's number was at 120—fifteen times what we believe is the highest acceptable amount!

Thankfully, with a solid detoxification program, Emily slowly came back to her old self. It took about a year—and some new plumbing and renovation in her home—but her brain fog has cleared. Once more, she's energetic, she's mentally astute, and she's awake enough every night to watch the eleven o'clock news (though we discourage everyone from watching the news before bed; the combination of stress and blue light is *not* a recipe for good sleep).

Before you start thinking Emily is a rare case, know that according to the CDC, there are 15.8 cases of lead poisoning per every 100,000 working adults.[9] Note: "100,000 working adults" means per 100,000 people working in companies that do blood lead testing as part of their OSHA requirements in states where it's mandated. In other words, the actual prevalence is most likely much higher.

And that's for lead *poisoning*. Now, as far as body burden goes, perhaps first we need to put a word in here that differentiates between poisoning and toxicity. The difference is that poisonings are often from overexposure within a short period of time, and the body is flooded beyond its ability to keep up and remove the toxins. The kids in Flint, Michigan, have lead poisoning from

9 "Adult Blood Lead Epidemiology and Surveillance—United States, 2008–2009," Centers for Disease Control and Prevention, July 1, 2011, www.cdc.gov/mmwr/preview/mmwrhtml/mm6025a2.htm.

their bad water. Their bodies literally cannot deal with the lead that they have been exposed to, and they are extremely ill as a result of it. Most of us, as adults, do not have lead *poisoning*. We have an *elevated toxic burden*—an elevated burden that stresses the whole body. That's the kind of people we deal with, the ones who have toxicities, not poisonings, and as you'll discover in Chapter 7, we do different kinds of testing to determine the toxic burden in our bodies.

But while lead is a serious contaminant in many people's water, it's not the only potential toxin we are unknowingly drinking.

> We have seen numerous clients who come in with mild cognitive impairment, exhibiting signs of dementia, and even having received a diagnosis of Alzheimer's. After a thorough exam, though, we often discover they have high levels of lead, mercury, and sometimes cadmium (particularly if they were smokers, cadmium will be more predominant). Thankfully, the damage is often reversible once the toxins are eliminated.

Tainted Water and Shameful Food

Let's face it. Our "clean" drinking water ain't so clean. Plenty of other industrial chemicals are keeping company with each other inside that perfectly clear liquid running from your taps. Here are just a few of the main culprits that could be wreaking havoc in our bodies.

Fluoride

"Look, Mom—no cavities!" That slogan was made famous in ads designed by Norman Rockwell for fluoride-enriched toothpaste back in the 1950s. But not everything about fluoride is so happy and positive. In fact, several countries, including Sweden, Germany, and Switzerland, have stopped putting fluoride in drinking water because it was deemed more harmful than beneficial.

I know what you're thinking! But we need fluoride for healthy teeth! That's what we are constantly told. I'm not going to go "there" with fluoride. But I will tell you *no one* should be ingesting it. First, do you know where the fluoride in our water comes from? Industrial sludge![10] Wonder what a Rockwell painting of *that* would look like!

The fluoride in our drinking water is actually an industrial by-product, which is a fancier term than *sludge*; it's an unprocessed leftover from fertilizer manufacturing. Right. Fertilizer. It's not good enough to be fertilizer, yet it's supposed to be good enough to go in our water.

But it's not. In fact, it's very, very bad for us. It's been associated with cognitive decline, hyperthyroidism, and poor absorption

---

10   Frank Zelko, "Toxic Treatment: The Story of Fluoride," Origins, https://origins.osu.edu/article/toxic-treatment-fluorides-transformation-industrial-waste-public-health-miracle.

of magnesium, calcium, and potassium, among other nutrients, and "population-based-studies strongly suggest that chronic fluoride ingestion is a possible cause of uterine cancer and bladder cancer; there may be a link with osteosarcoma."[11]

> **Fluoride did sh*t for me. I wound up with tons of cavities regardless of good dental hygiene. So I wound up with amalgam fillings, which is a great source for mercury!**

Mercury

Liquid mercury is a neurotoxin. It's also extraordinarily beautiful to look at. That's why I was playing with it back in high school. A thermometer broke, and beautiful balls of the silvery liquid bounced around. I just couldn't resist playing with them. They felt heavy and liquidy, but for some reason they didn't feel wet. Had I known the long-term consequences...well, anyway. It's bad for you. Really bad for you. It's bad for you to breathe in the vapors of it, which is one way you become toxic from amalgam fillings. It slowly vaporizes in your mouth, and you inhale

---

11 Stephen Peckham and Niyi Awofeso, "Water Fluoridation: A Critical Review of the Physiological Effects of Ingested Fluoride as a Public Health Intervention," *The Scientific World Journal* (2014), www.ncbi.nlm.nih.gov/pmc/articles/PMC3956646/.

those vapors.[12] It's bad for you when it gets absorbed into your skin. And it's bad for you to eat.

The primary source of mercury in food is fish. So you may be wondering how fish get exposed to it. After all, fish mothers lay eggs and abandon their babies; they don't hang around with a tub of Vicks VapoRub and a mercury-filled thermometer on hand for when their little ones are too sick to go to school. Fish get it because of us—we humans with our factories spewing heavy metal contaminants out into the air. Those contaminants eventually fall to the ground and get washed into our streams, rivers, and oceans. The contaminants get ingested every time a fish opens its mouth, and it goes in and out of their bodies as the water washes through their gills.

Little fish eat and ingest mercury. They are then eaten by bigger fish, which already have mercury from having eaten a lot of littler fish. Then those bigger fish are subsequently eaten by even larger fish, with their own burden, and so on. In that way, the mercury gets compounded in each bigger fish the further up the marine-life food chain you go. At the top of that chain, you have big fish like tuna, swordfish, mahi-mahi, shark, striped bass, and king mackerel who now have what is called "bio-accumulated" levels of mercury—meaning all the mercury from the tiny fish on up is in them. As you now know after reading Chapter 2, toxins get stored in the fat. So when people eat that delicious fatty tuna sushi, they are getting a side of mercury tossed in with it.

---

12 "Dental Amalgam Fillings," US Food and Drug Administration, https://www.fda.gov/medical-devices/dental-devices/dental-amalgam-fillings#:~:text=The%20form%20of%20mercury%20associated,mainly%20absorbed%20by%20the%20lungs

Aside from fish, there is another food out there that has a surprising amount of mercury in it. That food is corn syrup. Yes, corn syrup—high-fructose corn syrup, normal corn syrup, it doesn't matter. As reported back in 2009 in *Environmental Health*, mercury from corn syrup is in some very popular foods; a few of them, like Quaker Oatmeal to Go bars or Nutri-Grain strawberry cereal bars, even sound as if they might be good for you.[13] But don't let *any* name of *any* product fool you. Look at the ingredients and steer clear of corn syrup in any format!

The FDA hasn't really taken a stand (yet) on how much mercury should be allowed in corn syrup (we think the answer is *none*) but they did issue guidelines of what they consider "safe" levels of mercury in fish.[14] However, they are not looking at it in terms of individuals in the twenty-first century with chronic stress and other potential toxins in their lives. What's safe for one person may not be safe for you.

Plastics

In Chapter 2, you learned that when plastics are heated in a microwave, it can cause chemicals to leach into your food. What we didn't mention is where those chemicals come from

---

13   Renee Dufault, Blaise LeBlanc, Roseanne Schnoll, Charles Cornett, Laura Schweitzer, David Wallinga, Jane Hightower, Lyn Patrick, and Walter J. Lukiw, "Mercury from Chlor-alkali Plants: Measured Concentrations in Food Product Sugar," *Environmental Health* 8, no. 2 (2009), https://ehjournal.biomedcentral. com/track/pdf/10.1186/1476-069X-8-2.pdf; David Wallinga, Janelle Sorensen, Pooja Mottl, and Brian Yablon, *Not So Sweet: Missing Mercury and High Fructose Corn Syrup* (Minneapolis: Institute for Agriculture and Trade Policy, 2009), https://www. iatp.org/sites/default/files/421_2_105026.pdf.

14   "Advice about Eating Fish," US Food and Drug Administration, https://www.fda. gov/media/102331/download.

or why they're bad for your health. In short, plastics are petroleum by-products. They are made from natural gas and oil (and sometimes plants) that are turned into ethane and propane.[15] Those gases are then heated and processed to turn them into something called ethylene and propylene, and then a bunch of other stuff happens, which is beyond the scope of this book. The key takeaway here is that your plastic bowls, plates, water bottles, *baby bottles*, and everything else that's plastic is most likely a petroleum by-product.

Now, if you take nothing else from this book, at least take this: if something is a by-product of something else, it's generally *not* a good thing! And that's especially true with plastic. As it gets heated and melts, all the unnatural chemicals that went into making it are released. The result of that is that it's estimated *every human on the planet* has some plastic in their body (note that it's not just every human in Hollywood!), and it's believed the average American consumes more than seventy thousand microparticles of plastic a year![16] You know all those hot soups in the cylindrical plastic containers at the deli? Yeah, that plastic melted into your matzo balls. Ever see a Styrofoam container look a little wilted when your delivery arrives? Yep, that container melted into your chicken wings.

---

15   "How Are Plastics Made?" This Is Plastics, January 6, 2020, https://thisisplastics.com/plastics-101/how-are-plastics-made/.

16   Kieran D. Cox, Garth A. Covernton, Hailey L. Davies, John F. Dower, Francis Juanes, and Sarah E. Dudas, "Human Consumption of Microplastics," *Environmental Science & Technology* 53, no. 12 (2019): 7068–7074, doi:10.1021/acs.est.9b01517.

Can I Have a Side of Legos, Please?

Just how much plastic could you be consuming? Well... according to a 2019 study by WWF International, we are eating about two thousand tiny pieces of plastic a week. That is the equivalent of eating:[17]

- A plastic credit card each week

- A four-inch by two-inch Lego brick each month

- A fireman's helmet each year

- 5.5 pounds of plastic plumbing pipe each decade

And just because it's everywhere doesn't mean it's safe. Plastic in our bodies has been linked to a whole host of problems. It damages the central nervous system; irritates the mucus membranes of the eye, nose, and throat; creates muscle weakness; induces fatigue and nausea; causes birth defects; impairs your immune system; disrupts your endocrine system; and can

---

17 "Revealed: Plastic Ingestion by People Could Be Equating to a Credit Card a Week," WWF, June 12, 2019, https://wwf.panda.org/wwf_news/press_releases/?348337%2FRevealed-plastic-ingestion-by-people-could-be-equating-to-a-credit-card-a-week; Matthew Stock, "How Much Plastic Are You Eating?" Reuters, December 11, 2020, https://widerimage.reuters.com/story/how-much-plastic-are-you-eating.

cause cancer.[18] This is beginning to sound like the side effects listed at the end of a commercial for a pharmaceutical product, right? The crazy thing is, there's more!

You may have already stopped drinking from plastic water bottles or only use products that are labeled BPA-free. If so, that's a great first step, but it's not all you need to be aware of. PVC is just as bad for us and, unfortunately, it is used to contain food and drink products even though it will leach dioxins, phthalates, vinyl chloride, ethylene dichloride, lead, cadmium, and many other chemicals into your food!

A couple of recent *New York Times* articles are devoted to plastics and their toxins—in particular to phthalates. According to the research reported in those articles, phthalates can interfere and cause problems with just about every hormone in our body, but "the reproductive system in particular is extremely sensitive" to them. It's believed that a female exposed to phthalates in the womb may be predisposed to have fertility problems once she grows into an adult.[19] Baby boys don't fare any better. Early exposure to phthalates either in the womb or in early childhood is linked with lower testosterone levels.[20]

In Chapter 1, you read about what phthalates and lead will do to you. Here's a dirty laundry list of the potential impact of the other toxins:

18 Richard Harth, "Perils of Plastics: Risks to Human Health and the Environment," Arizona State University, March 18, 2010, https://biodesign.asu.edu/news/perils-plastics-risks-human-health-and-environment.

19 Liza Gross, "This Chemical Can Impair Fertility, but It's Hard to Avoid," New York Times, August 25, 2020, www.nytimes.com/2020/08/25/parenting/fertility-pregnancy-phthalates-toxic-chemicals.html.

20 Alice Callahan, "The Types of Plastics Families Should Avoid," New York Times, April 17, 2020, www.nytimes.com/article/plastics-to-avoid.html.

- **Dioxins:** damage the immune system, are endocrine disruptors, cause reproductive problems, cause developmental problems, and may cause cancer

- **Vinyl chloride:** irritates mucous membranes and respiratory tract, can damage the liver or cause liver cancer, and can result in neurological and behavioral alterations

- **Ethylene dichloride:** damages the nervous system, liver, and kidneys, and can cause respiratory distress and cardiac arrhythmia, nausea, and vomiting

- **Cadmium:** causes urinary, cardiovascular, and urinary tract damage, develops respiratory symptoms, and may lead to cancer in organs

See why PVC and plastics are just not good for us? To keep your exposure to PVC at a minimum, look for the recycle symbol on your plastic packaging. If the number 3 is listed with it, that means it has PVC. Don't buy it!

Perchlorate

Perchlorate is a natural chemical, which almost sounds as if it would be safe. It's natural, right? Just remember, the killer herb belladonna is also natural, as are arsenic and rattlesnake poison. Well, perchlorate can be added to that list of natural toxins. It is *extremely* water-soluble, so it easily filters into groundwater and drinking water. And it is found naturally in the ground in desert areas in the US. But don't think because you live someplace where it rains a lot that it can't impact you.

Perchlorate gets into our water supplies from a couple of sources. One is bleach; yes, the stuff we put in our washing machines. And the other is that it is used in the production of rocket fuel and, consequently, water supplies near facilities where rocket fuel is made tend to have higher levels of it. Do you know where rocket fuel is made? Neither do I. But I do know that I live in a suburban area in Massachusetts, and my lab results came back saying my perchlorate levels were off the charts. Seriously. The ninety-fifth percentile is a level of eleven. Mine was three times that, at thirty-one! I pride myself on being an overachiever, but this is one way I'm not proud of exceeding the set limits!

Artificial Colors, Flavors, and Sweeteners

Not many people are aware of this, but most of the artificial colors and flavors in our foods are just like plastics—they are derived from petroleum products. Because it seems so far-fetched, let me be clear. This stuff comes from the petroleum we fuel our cars with. Yes, that's in many of the artificial colors and flavors in our foods!

Artificial sweeteners, while not made from petroleum, are still not good for you. Some have even been linked to being carcinogenic. But even if they are perfectly safe cancer-wise, what you need to know is that artificial sweeteners can actually make you fat. It's not quite cast in stone, and the research is ongoing, but it's believed that simply tasting the artificial sweeteners tricks your body into thinking it's about to eat real sugar. So, with that first taste, your body gives a heads-up to your pancreas: "Hey, peeps! Sugar is coming! Put some insulin out!"

Your pancreas does what it's told, but when there is no sugar intake to match the preparatory insulin spike that's now coursing through your body, something else has to happen so you don't become hypoglycemic and pass out. The thing that happens is that you crave sugar and then you eat some carbs. And that explains why most people who drink a lot of artificially sweetened drinks wind up about ten pounds heavier than they were before they started using them.

Glyphosate

Most of our grains are genetically modified so that they can be more easily grown on monocrop farms. Monocrops are preferable for large industrial farms because they can use only one kind of seed and then manage the maintenance of the plants in only one particular way. As you can see, that results in a more efficient way of farming than having a variety of crops where each has a particular need for water, fertilizer, or other care.

However, Mother Nature never thought a monocrop was a good idea. She's like, "If you want only one kind of plant to grow someplace, put it in a pot and set it on your windowsill!" That's why it's so hard to create a weed-free lawn—it goes against what Mother Nature designed.

Genetically modifying our grains is one way to bypass the difficulty of developing a monocrop. Now they've developed wheat, corn, and other grains to tolerate being sprayed with Roundup and other weed killers, the key ingredient of which is glyphosate. On the surface, that seems like a good idea. You kill all the bad weeds, and your good crop of grain thrives. That's a win-win for the farmer and the plant. However, it's a win-win-lose when you add in the consumer, because when you eat those plants, it turns out you're eating glyphosate.

Perhaps an even worse use of glyphosate is in a practice called "browning," when entire fields are sprayed with eight to eleven times the amount of the herbicide regularly used. They do it to completely dry out an area.[21] Oh wait! We forgot an important part here: *they do it right before harvesting the crops!* Particularly non-GMO crops! Wheat and other grains and legumes are perfect targets for this practice, which is one of the reasons why Cheerios and other cereals have glyphosate in them. It's so bad that every single garbanzo bean (chickpea) tested in the United States and Canada so far has been found to have glyphosate residue.[22]

So, yes, glyphosate is everywhere! It's in your hummus and probably the pita chips too. It's in the buns you have with your Fourth of July cheeseburgers, the pizza you ate from the great Italian place down the street, that heart-healthy box of Cheerios you feed to your children! And don't forget your oatmeal!

The only way you can get around eating glyphosate is by eating organic vegetables and fruit, and if you eat meats, you should choose from animals that ate organic grains because animals, it turns out, are loaded with glyphosate too. Sounds like an expensive pain in the a**, I know, but trust me. You want to stay clear of this chemical. Because when you eat it, you are eating

---

21   Ken Roseboro, "Why Is Glyphosate Sprayed on Crops Right before Harvest?" EcoWatch, January 25, 2021, www.ecowatch.com/roundup-cancer-1882187755.html.

22   "The Concerns about Glyphosate Residue in Food," FoodPrint, November 4, 2020, https://foodprint.org/blog/glyphosate-residue-in-food/.

a carcinogen, which in the long run could be more expensive than your organic broccoli.[23] By the way, even organic items are sometimes cross-contaminated with glyphosate since they're grown near crops that have been sprayed with Roundup. Truly, no good deed goes unpunished!

Not-So-Fun Fact: Your Kale Might Be Bad for You!

Organic broccoli, cauliflower, kale, and other greens from California are often loaded with thallium, a heavy metal considered to be one of the most dangerous to the human body. Why? Because it damages the mitochondria of cells and displaces potassium. Oh, wait! Were you asking why do organic veggies from California have such a dangerous heavy metal? Because the soil is contaminated with it in many areas due to fracking and other industrialized processes.

Cancers linked to glyphosate include non-Hodgkin's lymphoma, renal tubule carcinoma, pancreatic islet cell adenoma, and skin tumors. There are also studies that indicate glyphosate disrupts the gut microbiome, which is where all the work is done to digest your food.

---

23 "IARC Monograph on Glyphosate," International Agency for Research on Cancer, https://www.iarc.fr/featured-news/media-centre-iarc-news-glyphosate/.

Keep that word—microbiome—in mind. Part of getting clean and staying clean requires you to make your microbiome as healthy as possible. But before we talk about fixing things and detoxing, let's finish talking about from where we're getting all these toxins in the first place.

But organic foods cost more! We hear that all the time. And yes, they do. However, the up-front cost of organic food is a known amount you can see on your grocery receipt. Whereas people like me, people who are sensitive to toxins, have no idea what the long-term medical expenses will be to get rid of the toxins from conventionally grown produce. Nor do we know how our quality of life will be impacted by them. So you have a choice: pay the piper now, or pay him later, which will most likely be more expensive.

Are you beginning to wonder if your diet is healthy enough? Don't worry. We have plenty of guidelines to help you choose the foods that are least likely to be toxic and provide a punch of nutrition later, in Chapter 9.

Moving from the Inside to the Outside

Now that you have a good concept of how the food and drinks you put inside your body can make you toxic, you might be wondering what to do about them. Don't worry. We won't leave you hanging. After we discuss all the potential pathways toxins take to come to you, we'll spend a few chapters on how to make them leave. And we're almost there.

Right now, though, we need to move from what goes into us that makes us toxic to what's outside of us that's making us toxic. So let's see just how dirty our homes, wardrobe, and environment are.

Hot Top Tips

1. Say no to plastics as much as possible—that includes home storage bowls. Use wooden or silicone products for baby toys. And that vinyl shower curtain you never liked to begin with? What better reason to be done with it?

2. Your municipal water supplier should be able to provide a report on the safety of your drinking water. Find it. Read it. Filter your water if you're concerned!

3. Start reading ingredients on food labels. Better yet, stop eating food with labels!

4. Try to eat organic fruits, veggies, and grains (small amounts!), and choose flesh proteins from animals fed an organic diet.

5. Avoid the high-mercury fish and artificial colors,
   flavors, and preservatives

CHAPTER 4

Deceptive Beauty

I used to think I had chemical sensitivities. I couldn't stand walking down the laundry supply aisles of the supermarket, and whenever I was in a department store and one of those nice perfume ladies would start walking toward me, I'd run in the opposite direction. I just couldn't tolerate the smells. I'd get headaches and even feel a little nauseous. My poor mother-in-law! I made her stop wearing perfume when she came to our house since I used to get so sick!

After I ran the mold test and started detoxing to get the mold numbers down, I realized those things didn't bother me as much. It was an eye-opener for me, as I never realized the chemical sensitivities were signs that toxins were building up in my body. With twenty-twenty hindsight, though, I see it now: those supermarket detergents and cleaning supplies, and the perfumes those women in the cosmetics departments were spraying, were all chemicals, toxic chemicals my body wasn't willing to tolerate.

Chapter 9 opens with a before and after of my lab test. As you'll see, I was pretty loaded! That's because environmental toxins are insidious. We're absorbing them from literally everywhere and everything. Case in point: here is some of the sh*t that showed up in my first toxicity panel, where it came from, and the potential harm it can do.

TOXIN	SOURCE	HARM
Monoethylphthalate (MEP)	**Bath and beauty products, cosmetics, perfumes,** oral pharmaceuticals, insect repellants, **adhesives, inks, varnishes**	Implicated in reproductive damage, lowers testosterone, and alters sexual development in children; depresses leukocyte (white blood cell) function; and causes cancer.
2-3-4 methylhippuric acid (2,-3-,4-MHA)	Paints, lacquers, pesticides, cleaning fluids, fuel and exhaust fumes, **perfumes,** insect repellents	Results in nausea, vomiting, dizziness, central nervous system depression, and death(!).
Diphenyl phosphate (DPP)	Plastics, electronic equipment, **nail polish,** resins	Causes endocrine disruption and is linked to reproductive and developmental problems.

Note how some of the sources are in bold? Something I don't think many people are aware of is that our personal care products are often loaded with toxins, particularly ones that are endocrine disruptors. (I used to take great pride in how nice my nails looked and painted them a different color every week!

Now? Ummm...yeah, natural nails it is! But the upside is that, as I've cleared these toxins, my nails have actually gotten stronger and break less often!)

Endo What?

The phrase *endocrine disruptors* often appears when anyone talks about toxins and their effects on the body. It may not sound like much; I mean, a disruptor? Whatever! We've all had disrupted sleep, right? We just tell the hubs to roll over so he quits snoring and then nod back off. However, it's not so simple when it comes to the endocrine system.

Your endocrine system is the management company of your hormones. All your hormones. And for each one you have, there is another hormone that balances it out. Remember when we spoke in Chapter 2 about cortisol? The hormone dehydroepi-androsterone (DHEA) goes up when cortisol goes down. DHEA is something that helps us relax and de-stress (among other things). That's why you cannot have high levels of both cortisol and DHEA at the same time. Nor can you have low levels at the same time. All hormones work that way if nothing interferes with them.

However, some toxic chemicals can mimic a hormone, so your body thinks that hormone is acting, which means the balancing one must be lowered (or raised, depending on what that action is). Other toxins just prevent a hormone from being used, so the other one is left sitting by the phone, waiting for it to ring.

Regardless of which way they disrupt, when toxins get involved with your hormones, all h*ll breaks loose. Anything from learning disabilities in children to reproductive problems in adults can happen, as well as birth defects, cancers, and a whole host of autoimmune diseases.

In short, it's not as simple to fix an endocrine disruption as it is to roll over and go back to sleep. That's why it's imperative to have as little exposure to those toxins as possible. We will go into just how to limit your exposure in Chapter 9. Right now, we're just going to discuss where a lot of these toxins come from and how they get into our bodies.

We Are All Thin-Skinned

Our skin does a great job of keeping our insides on the inside, but it works like a one-way street when it comes to the outside. That might seem like common sense, right? I mean we put on hand lotion and *rub it in*. It doesn't stay on the top, outside of us.

Think about that.

You pump out a dollop of lotion and rub it into your skin. Sure, it's making the outside soft and supple. We all like that. But look at the ingredients of your lotion. *That's* what's going into your body. Your bloodstream says hello to the ingredients and, when it finds one that's a toxin, it hurries it away to the liver. If the liver is too busy or overloaded, it takes that toxin to a fat cell. This is one of the reasons it's difficult to lose fat when your body is stressed or overtaxed; the body needs the fat cells to store the toxins you're not eliminating.

Before you start thinking thoughts like *Surely, there's nothing that bad in my lotion! There are laws against that, aren't there?* let me assure you that surely there are plenty of bad things that could be in your lotions—your shampoos, your conditioners, makeup, and all your other personal care products too—as well as in the clothing you're wearing, the furniture you're sitting on, and just about anything that comes in contact with your skin. And very few laws address them.

So let's dive into this a little to see what we need to look for and what we can do about it.

Personal Care Products

It's been estimated that after the average American in the twenty-first century showers and gets ready to go to work in the morning, that person has been exposed to more than a *hundred* different chemicals from their bodywash or soap, shampoo, conditioner, hairstyling products, deodorants, and cosmetics. OMFG.

Meanwhile, the law that regulates what manufacturers can put in their products was last updated in 1938.[24] For real? That's crazy! The world was a completely different place back then, and we have tons more chemicals now! Not only that, but there are so many loopholes in that law that companies can create their own interpretation of words like *organic, natural,* and *hospital-approved.* And they can use the word *fragrance* to mean anything. Seriously. If they have a proprietary formula they don't want anyone to know, they just list "fragrance" on their ingredients, and they've got their legal bases covered.

---

24 Amy Roeder, "Harmful, Untested Chemicals Rife in Personal Care Products," Harvard School of Public Health, February 13, 2014, www.hsph.harvard.edu/news/features/harmful-chemicals-in-personal-care-products.

Obviously, it's really hard to protect yourself from toxins if you don't know there are toxins in something! The easy work-around to that is to read an ingredient label, and if you don't recognize a word—or it's a word with thirty syllables and a couple of numbers—don't buy it. Don't rub it into your skin. And definitely don't wash your hair with it or line your lips with it.

Another easy way is to check out one of our favorite resources, the Environmental Working Group (EWG) (www.ewg.org). Their research is enormous and covers personal care products as well as common house and home chemicals in things like cleaners and detergents.

They have a list of twelve chemicals that they call the Toxic Twelve, which you should always avoid as best you can. They include:

- **Formaldehyde:** an endocrine disruptor and known carcinogen

- **Paraformaldehyde:** a type of formaldehyde

- **Methylene glycol:** another type of formaldehyde

- **Quaternium-15:** something that releases formaldehyde

- **Mercury:** a heavy metal that can damage the kidneys and nervous system

- **Dibutyl and diethylhexyl phthalates:** endocrine disruptors, particularly damaging to the reproductive system

- **Isobutyl and isopropyl parabens:** endocrine disruptors, also particularly damaging to the reproductive system

- **The long-chain per- and polyfluoroalkyl substances known as PFAS:** chemicals that are linked to cancer

- **M- and o-Phenylenediamine, used in hair dyes:** an irritant that sensitizes the skin, damages DNA, and can cause cancer

Remember this for your next trivia night: in the seventeenth and eighteenth century in England, hat makers were often exposed to mercury vapors from the felting process they used to form hats from wool. Because so many in their industry suffered mental illness as a consequence of mercury exposure, the phrase *mad as a hatter* was coined.

While you're thinking about overhauling your cosmetic counter, do know that's just the tip of the iceberg for objects in your personal world that could make you sick. Our clothing, furniture, and the stuff we use to maintain a happy home are just as toxic.

Here's another snapshot of my toxic profile.

TOXIN	SOURCE	HARM
Phenylglyoxylic acid (PGO)	Plastics, building materials, car exhaust, and food packaging	Impacts the central nervous system; causes concentration problems, muscle weakness, fatigue, and nausea; mucous membrane irritant.
N-acetyl phenyl cysteine (NAP)	Vehicle exhaust, cigarette smoke, off-gassing from synthetic materials	A mutagenic and carcinogenic; can cause nausea, vomiting, dizziness, lack of coordination, central nervous system depression, hematological abnormalities, and death.
N-acetyl (2-cyanoethyl) cysteine (NACE)	Acrylic fibers, resins, rubber	Causes headaches, dizziness, fatigue, chest pain; the EU has classified it as a carcinogen.

I got "lucky" with these particular toxins, as they are barely present in my profile. However, many of my patients have not had the same fortune. Why? Look at the ones listed in bold: plastics, building materials, synthetic materials, and acrylic fibers. That's stuff in our homes, in our furniture and clothing! Here are some potential avenues of exposure.

Clothing

You know that new-clothes smell, don't you? It's super toxic. Often textile manufacturers will treat fabrics with formaldehyde, and, to make matters worse, clothing manufacturers will layer chemicals on top of that to hide the formaldehyde smell or make the clothing smell better. This is why you really *should* wash your new clothes prior to wearing them. Maybe wash them a few times.

What about the dry-clean-only stuff? Well, taking it to the dry cleaner before wearing it might just add dry-cleaner chemicals onto it, including perchloroethylene, a carcinogen that has been outlawed in California because it's so toxic, and N-acetyl (propyl)cysteine (NAPR), which is a reproductive toxin that can also cause sensory and motor deficits, decreased cognitive function, and central nervous system impairment. So look for an organic dry cleaner and ask them what they use that's so safe. If they really *are* an organic cleaner, they will use a silicone-based solvent or a carbon-based one, like hydrocarbon and/or carbon dioxide (CO_2).

If you don't have an organic dry cleaner near you, we suggest you air those clothes out for several days. Don't hang them in your closet, packed tightly between your favorite sweater and those slacks that make your rear look great. Hang them where the open air can help dissipate and off-gas the chemicals. And, honestly, I've found that many clothes that say "dry-clean only" do quite fine when washed on the gentle cycle and hung up to dry! Obviously, you'll have to iron them, which isn't so fun!

What is off-gassing? Basically, it's chemical vapors escaping products and contaminating the air—thus contaminating you, too, when you breathe it in or your skin comes in contact with it. And off-gassing isn't restricted to clothing, as you'll discover in the next chapter. It happens with furniture, mattresses, finished floors, drapery, and anything that uses glues, paints, and varnishes. Basically, if something has a chemical smell to it, it's off-gassing.

Something else to think about regarding your clothing is to see what it is made from. Note that two of the toxins above are found in common textiles made with synthetic fabrics and acrylic fibers. Perhaps it's not a surprise to you by now that many of our synthetic and acrylic products are petroleum-based products. That includes nylon, spandex, Lycra, acrylics, and rayon—think about it: they are all just a few molecules away from being hard plastics!

Some people are so reactive to these fabrics that no amount of washing will be of help to them. For the rest of us, the better our bodies can detox, the more likely we can wear these clothes with no problems.

Of course, what you put on your body is only part of the equation. Your ambient environment is filled with invisible dangers from toxins that can also cross the skin barrier as well as be inhaled and even eaten.

Hot Top Tips

1. Visit EWG's website and use their Skin Deep reports to evaluate how safe your personal care products currently are.

2. Wash all your brand-new clothes.

3. I don't care how well your dry cleaner protects the
   buttons on your blouses; find a new one if they
   aren't organic.

CHAPTER 5

The Invisible Dangers

One of my long-term patients is a teacher. For a while, we'd been working on symptoms that we believed were related to mold, but we couldn't quite pinpoint her exposure. It just wouldn't go away. Sometimes, it would clear up over the summer, but not completely. So we knew mold was present and growing in a hidden space somewhere in her life on a regular basis. We weren't sure if it eased up in the summer because she was outside more in general, or if there was another reason.

Results from air quality tests in her home came back negative for mold, though, so it wasn't coming from there. I suspected it was from the school where she worked. Just for the record, for some reason a lot of schools and dorms are moldy! Every September, though, after a three-month break from being in the school building, I'd ask her if she felt worse than she did over the summer. She always said no. Until September 2020.

In 2020, she said yes. Why was it so different? Well...the pandemic had closed her school down the previous March, so she had six months to fully recover from her mold exposure at school, a length of time she never had before. Being at home also provided her the opportunity to focus on fully doing her mold treatments in a way that she struggled with when she worked at the school full-time. That added treatment, along with the time out of the building, gave her long enough to remove significantly more of the mold toxins from her body, so she was feeling great by the time September rolled around. But when she had to enter that building for a few days a week, her symptoms started up again.

Mold is just one of the invisible dangers in the world around us. And I suspect mold has always been a problem for humanity. Think about it: before we had central heating and air conditioning, our homes were often described as dank and drafty, particularly in older books. But now that we do have central heating and air conditioning, we also have homes that are more airtight to keep the temperature where we want it. That makes for energy savings and lower utility bills, but it also means the toxins that mold releases are kept inside our buildings as well. They cannot dissipate on a breeze, so they become more concentrated in the air we breathe while we're inside. And remember that rain-barrel analogy from Chapter 2—our bodies can only deal with so much. A regular exposure to mold toxins every day at work or at home can fill up our barrel and become too much for our liver and other systems to handle. That's when we start experiencing symptoms.

If you only had mold for your liver to detox, *and* you didn't have the stress that you do now, *and* you slept more because there were no glowing screens to entertain you at night, *and* you moved your body more because there was little time to just sit around, *and* your food wasn't nearly as contaminated or moldy, *then* you would probably deal with the mold pretty well. Your body wouldn't be overflowing its rain barrel.

Or, possibly, mold explains why so many women had headaches and men were described as phlegmy in the Victorian era. Regardless, it's a problem for many people now, and as with most environmental toxins, it can be hard to figure out just where the exposure is coming from. The toxins are literally everywhere. So addressing mold means you take a multi-pronged approach, as you would with other toxins, and deal with it based on the person's genetics, exposure, and lifestyle (which you'll learn about in this chapter of the book). The fact that my patient felt better when she was not in the school was a huge clue for us about where the exposure could be coming from, and it served as a great starting point for us to help her.

An Inspiration!

When Lana came to me for an evaluation, she was suffering from a wide range of complaints, including dizziness, vertigo, joint pains, weight gain, extreme fatigue and exercise intolerance, headaches, sleep disruptions, and brain fog.

A thorough workup on her revealed she had Lyme, Babesia, and Bartonella (the latter two are bacterial infections you can get from ticks and other sources). She also tested positive for mycotoxin toxicities and had an elevated body burden of lead and mercury.

We've been working on her health for *two* years, peeling away and treating each of these issues. But the treatment is working.

She's now off the Lyme/Bartonella/Babesia treatment, is rid of her metals, has very low levels of environmental toxins, and is wrapping up her mold treatment (down to two strains from six).

And she's beginning to feel amazing—beginning to; she's not quite there yet. There's no more dizziness, brain fog, headaches, or joint pain. Her sleep has improved, and she's getting more and a better quality of sleep, and there's been a great improvement in her energy levels.

She's so inspiring! She worked extremely hard to get better and is now clearly seeing the impact!

It's in the Air Tonight

If you feel bad at home and feel better when you're elsewhere for a couple of days, then it's very possible your home is making you sick. Of course, the same can be said for your workplace too. Regardless, paying close attention to your symptoms to see if they wax and wane in response to your location can help point you in the direction of the source of your struggles.

Frequently, it's the new things in our lives that are the most toxic. That new smell of your car, carpeting, sofa, mattress, or other item frequently has the same source as your new-clothing smell: formaldehyde. But there are also flame retardants, fungicides, insecticides, and herbicides off-gassing from those items as well.

> **Ever walk into a clothing store at the beginning of summer to be bombarded by that rubbery smell from their cute flip-flops? Those shoes are off-gassing! Turn around and go someplace else!**

How can you tell if something is off-gassing? It has a chemical smell. It's that simple. After something is given a chance to air out long enough, often the smell will be gone and it will be safe to bring into your home.

Otherwise, if at all possible, try to leave whatever is off-gassing outside your home until the smell is gone. And if it must come inside, leave it in a place where you don't frequent and open the windows as much as possible.

Mattresses, in particular, need *a lot* of time to off-gas. In addition to formaldehyde, mattresses off-gas these dangerous chemicals:

- **Toluene:** associated with central nervous system ailments that run the gamut from headaches to hallucinations to comas, arrhythmias, depressed respiratory functions, nausea, and electrolyte imbalances

- **Chlorofluorocarbons (CFCs):** connected with reduced coordination, headaches, and lightheadedness, and at high enough concentration they can disrupt heart rhythms

- **Benzene:** can decrease red blood cells, which may lead to anemia, cause problems with bone marrow, and weaken the immune system

- **Trichloroethane:** causes central nervous system problems including headaches, dizziness, poor coordination, and even coma; may cause hypotension and cardiac dysrhythmia

Unfortunately, when it comes to mattresses (and furniture, draperies, other upholstered products, and some clothing), there is yet another potential toxin we need to discuss: flame retardants, which don't just off-gas. They can leach into your body and be absorbed into your skin.

Flame Retardants

We mentioned why flame retardants were invented, and we're all for safety and protecting people from house fires. So, we get it: flame retardants on furniture, window blinds, and mattresses were created out of concern for people's well-being. Unfortunately, the chemicals that are in those flame retardants come with nasty side effects.

While there are numerous brands of fire retardants created for industrial use, most can be broken down into one of two categories: brominated or organophosphorus.

Brominated flame retardants are based on a bunch of dangerous toxins:

- **Polybrominated diphenyl ethers (PBDEs):** These guys are a little extra evil because they are made not to bond to the products they are applied to. That means when they are applied to furniture, they are easily released into the air. While most research has been on the negative effect PBDEs can cause on children, which includes everything from low birth weight to smaller size and impaired neurological development,[25] some animal studies are connecting them to cancer.

- **Tetrabromobisphenol A (TBBPA):** This toxic chemical is used in electronics, paper, and other textiles, and it happens to be the most popular flame retardant used. It's so popular, in fact, that it's been found everywhere: in dust, soil, water, fish, and...um...human tissues. Which is a very bad thing, indeed. The National

---

25 National Toxicology Program, *NTP Technical Report on the Toxicology Studies of a Pentabromodiphenyl Ether Mixture* (Research Triangle Park, NC: US Department of Health and Human Services, 2016), https://ntp.niehs.nih.gov/ntp/htdocs/lt_rpts/tr589_508.pdf.

Toxicology Program (managed by the US Department of Health and Human Services) did a study on this flame retardant in mice and concluded that it caused uterine cancer in female rats and liver cancer in male rats.[26]

- **Hexabromocyclododecane (HBCD):** This chemical isn't found in mattresses or soft furnishings much, but it is found in building materials, where there is a risk for it to leach out into the air and get into indoor dust, which we then breathe and even eat. It's an endocrine disruptor and it also negatively impacts the brain.

You may be terrified of flame retardants at this point, but we still have another group to look at. Those are the organophosphorus flame retardants. They are new in the world of flame retardants and have actually been invented as alternatives to replace the older ones deemed too dangerous. However, no one has deemed these new guys safe yet. In fact, the National Toxicology Program is studying them now, and early results are showing they aren't much better.[27] (Don't worry; in Chapter 9 we'll talk about all the specific steps you can take to avoid your exposure to flame retardants and how to find safe alternatives for your mattresses.)

---

26 National Toxicology Program, *NTP Technical Report on the Toxicology Studies of Tetrabromobisphenol A* (Research Triangle Park, NC: US Department of Health and Human Services, 2014), https://ntp.niehs.nih.gov/ntp/htdocs/lt_rpts/tr587_508.pdf

27 The National Toxicology Program is a department within the US Department of Health and Human Services.

Mold

Possibly on the opposite end of the toxic chemical spectrum from flame retardants is mold. Whereas flame retardants are concerned with potential fires, are often on new things, and are man-made, mold is concerned with water, is typically (but not always) associated with established or older things, and is a natural occurrence.

Mold loves to invade places that are exposed to water or that stay damp and warm. As such, it is a potential danger for any building that has been flooded or has had some kind of water damage. So if your drywall gets soaked through when the hose to your washing machine bursts, mold can easily thrive and grow out of sight on the wood inside your walls. It prefers places that are somewhat porous, so paper or cardboard products, ceiling tiles, wood, insulation, drywall, carpet, and upholstery are all excellent homes for mold.

But it will make do with a smooth surface if it has to. Which is why it grows in air ducts when people get humidifiers to attach to their heating systems.

Of course, the concern isn't the mold itself; it's the mold toxins. Mold puts out spores called mycotoxins, and different varieties of mold will produce different mycotoxins. Some strains are more toxic than others. And for people who have a heightened sensitivity to mold, they suffer when exposed to any, and with extended exposure, their suffering only increases (as experienced by my patient Lana as well as myself).

Symptoms from mold toxicity are similar to any other airborne allergy: headaches, stuffy nose, itchy eyes and skin, and worsening asthma. For people with ongoing exposure to large amounts of mold or who are highly sensitive to it, eczema, fever, and difficulty breathing are frequently indicated.

When we speak about mold, most of the time it's in reference to environmental mold—the stuff hiding in our attics, behind baseboards, above the ceiling tiles, and anyplace that is dark and humid. However, people who are sensitive to mold need to be aware that certain foods are prone to being moldy. In fact, some are not just prone to being moldy, they are always moldy!

If you think you may be sensitive to mold, you may want to remove the following from your diet:

- Alcohol made from grains

- Cheese

- Coffee

- Dried fruits and fruit juice

- Peanut butter

- Processed meats

- Wheat, barley, rice, maize

- Cereals

- Wine

- Peanuts and pistachios

- Leftover foods

As you can see, there is potential for toxins to come to you through just about everything. And if all that wasn't scary enough, there's one more thing we'd like to talk about: EMFs.

EMFs

I realize there are some controversies regarding whether EMFs (electromagnetic frequencies) cause harm to humans. The research is ongoing, so in the interim, I can only talk about what Ed and I have seen in our practice. And the fact is, we have helped patients who do suffer ill consequences from being exposed to EMFs.

If you think about it, it only makes sense that EMFs can have some kind of effect on us. Our bodies are biomagnetic, meaning we have a literal magnetic field around us. That's why MRI machines can see into our bodies. They use high-powered magnets to get the magnetic resonance of our cells and tissues.

Keep that in mind as you think about the changes in our electronics over the past couple of decades. We've all been increasingly exposed to and bombarded by EMFs from cell towers, high-tension wires, Wi-Fi, cell phones, and Bluetooth systems. For some people, when they become overburdened by EMFs from those products, they suffer brain fog, fatigue, insomnia, anxiety, muscle weakness, and poor muscle recovery after working out.

It's a tough thing to do, but the only way to know if you are someone who's sensitive to EMFs is to limit your exposure to them and see if you get better. Turn off your cell phones and Wi-Fi at night and see if that helps. Even better, go on a retreat far from cell towers or high-tension wires—preferably for a week or so—and monitor how you feel there compared to when you're back.

A place looking more and more attractive to me is Green Bank, West Virginia. Back in 1958, when the world's largest fully steerable radio telescope was built there, the national government established a thirteen-thousand-square-mile area around it as a radio-free zone. There are no Wi-Fi signals in the vicinity, and people within ten miles of the telescope cannot use any kind of Bluetooth device or a microwave, unless they are in something called a Faraday box, which blocks EMFs.

One other thing to be aware of is that as the world adopts 5G technology for broadband cellular networks, more people may become sensitive to EMFs. The radiation from 5G is much more than from 3G. It is believed to be a bigger problem for more people.

Again, if you feel better after you've been away from your home or work environment, that's one way of knowing if there's something in that place making you sick. Otherwise, you will have to do some testing and guessing when it comes to figuring out your level of exposure to toxins. Or have a consultation with a Functional Medicine provider for guidance. We love sleuthing this stuff out!

Tire Plastics

Off-gassing, mold, and EMFs you're probably familiar with. But have you thought about what your car tires are doing to you? Aside from taking you and your family everywhere you need to go?

Here's a little not-fun fact: our water, air, and soil are full of microparticles of plastics from—wait for it—tires! Who would have guessed? Not many. I mean, even *National Geographic* was surprised. They call tires "the plastic polluter you never thought about."[28]

Tires are made from rubber, a plastic polymer, and a bunch of other chemicals that probably aren't good for us either. The important one to note is the plastic polymer. Because as tires wear out, they flake off those plastic polymers, which end up in our rivers and oceans. Inevitably, they end up in our fish, and then they end up in our bodies.

If you think you're safe because you don't eat fish, you'll have to think twice. As long as you're breathing, you're exposed to plastic polymers from tires. The air pollution from them is estimated to be "a thousand times worse than car emissions"![29]

I'm particularly peeved by the tire issue. N-acetyl(3,4-dihydroxybutyl)cysteine (NADB) happens to be one of the toxins I had too much of in my system. It comes from synthetic rubber in tires and is a known carcinogen. It's also linked to cardiovascular disease. Grrrr.

28 Tik Root, "Tires: The Plastic Polluter You Never Thought About," National Geographic, May 3, 2021, www.nationalgeographic.com/environment/article/tires-unseen-plastic-polluter.

29 Rachel Evans, "Pollution from Tire Wear 1,000 Times Worse than Exhaust Emissions," *Tire Technology International*, March 11, 2020, www.tiretechnologyinternational.com/news/regulations/pollution-from-tire-wear-1000-times-worse-than-exhaust-emissions.html#:~:text=Air%20pollution%20from%20tire%20wear,problem%2C%20and%20is%20currently%20unregulated.&text=5%20and%2073%25%20of%20PM10.

Pesticides, Herbicides, and Fungicides

We don't have to define what these are to you; you probably already know. And you may even already suspect they can be harmful for you, which they are.

Your exposure to them comes from landscaping companies (or maybe even your spouse or partner) spraying them on yards, playgrounds, and in public spaces. They are everywhere. Granted, the pesticides are created to kill things much smaller than you, and the herbicides and fungicides are intended to kill plants and fungi. So, on the surface, it may seem hard to believe that they could pose a danger to you.

However, no one has done a study to see if chronic micro-doses of those chemicals over a series of years are dangerous. They have only done studies to see how much a healthy adult can tolerate in a one-time exposure. Before you start thinking along the lines of *What's the big deal? I'm not a plant! How can an herbicide hurt me?* remember that Agent Orange is a chemical created to be harmful to plants and it's causing dreadful harm to the children of adults who were exposed to it.[30]

For years, you can be bombarded with those toxins every day—they can be absorbed into your skin, breathed into your lungs, and eaten either in food sprayed with them or by accident because they are in the air around your meal. So, little by little,

---

30 George Black and Christopher Anderson, "The Victims of Agent Orange the US Has Never Acknowledged," *New York Times,* March 16, 2021, www.nytimes.com/2021/03/16/magazine/laos-agent-orange-vietnam-war.html?referringSource=articleShare.

every day, you're being dosed with toxins. Is it hard to fathom they could be dangerous to you?

It's not hard for me to fathom at all, especially since I had toxic levels in my body. My first lab results showed I was toxic with:

TOXIN	SOURCE	HARM
2,4-dichlorophenoxy-acetic acid (2-,4-D)	Common herbicide that was once an ingredient in Agent Orange	Associated with headaches, dizziness, peripheral neuropathy, seizures, impaired reflexes, and weakness. It is also a known endocrine disruptor.
Diethylphosphate (DEP)	Pesticide (It's an organophosphate, which is a group of toxins that are considered some of the most poisonous in the world.)	Causes overstimulation of nerve cells, diarrhea, abnormal behavior (including aggression and depression). Children born to exposed mothers have impaired reflexes. And children exposed to them are at double the normal risk of developing autism.
3-hydroxypropylmercap-turic acid (3-HPMA)	Herbicide	Associated with diabetes and insulin resistance.

Not only did I test positive for those three toxins, I tested as having elevated levels of them! Yet, guess what? I never used any of that stuff in my own yard, although I have zero clue what the landscapers used on my childhood lawn. That means I got them from foods I've eaten or from the rest of the world using them.

Cleaning Products

Finally, we'll end this chapter by talking a little about our cleaning products. Similar to our personal care products, many of our household cleaners have chemicals that have never been tested on us for their safety. Nor are there federal rules and regulations that they *must* be safe. And many of those chemicals are endocrine disruptors (you know, dangerously messing up your hormones, as we discussed in Chapter 2) and possible carcinogens.

If you look at the product labels for the things you store under your kitchen sink, you might notice that many of them carry warnings about their safety. "May be hazardous" some of them say. Others suggest you keep away from your eyes and that you don't breathe in the vapors. Still others say to use gloves and not let the cleaner contact your skin.

In addition to phthalates and perchloroethylene, which we've already highlighted in this book, here are a few other common concerning ingredients in your household cleaners:

- **Triclosan:** Frequently found in liquid dishwashing detergents and antibacterial hand soaps. A big worry here, and with most antibacterial products, is that it can encourage drug-resistant bacteria, which is a different concern than toxins. As a poison, though, it's a suspected endocrine disruptor and carcinogen.

- **Quaternary ammonium compounds:** Ingredients in fabric softeners and many cleaners labeled antibacterial.

These are also skin irritants (making their presence in
fabric softeners somewhat ironic), and they have caused
otherwise healthy people to develop asthma.

- **2-butoxyethanol:** A common solvent in glass and multi-
  purpose cleaners. This is a tricky one because, for some
  reason, it doesn't have to be listed on the label as an
  ingredient! However, it has a powerful "clean" smell that
  you'd probably recognize if you smelled it. But don't sniff
  too long! The inhaled vapors can cause liver and kidney
  damage and pulmonary edema.

- **Chlorine:** You know this one well: it's bleach. It's in
  toilet-bowl cleaners, mold and mildew removers, laundry products, and deep-cleaners. How many of us asso-
  ciate the smell of chlorine with that "fresh, clean" smell
  of our towels after they are bleached? It's scary because
  chlorine is especially wicked. It's not just a matter of
  either you breathing it in or it seeping in through your
  skin; it's dangerous in both ways. In addition to that, it's
  in many municipal water sources, where it reacts with
  carbon-containing compounds to form organochlorines
  that we drink in our water. Why is that such a terrible
  thing? Well, organochlorines contribute to hormone-re-
  lated conditions, cancer of male and female reproductive systems, developmental toxicity, neurotoxicity, and
  immunotoxicity.[31]

---

31 Gourounti Kleanthi, "Mechanisms of Actions and Health Effects of Organochlo-
rine Substances: A Review," *Health Science Journal* (2015), www.hsj.gr/medicine/
mechanisms-of-actions-and-health-effects-of-organochlorine-substances-a-re-
view.php?aid=3667.

- **Perchlorate:** We just talked about this in the last chapter but wanted to add something here. If you keep a bottle of bleach on hand for emergency laundry purposes or something, maybe consider getting rid of it. The crazy thing about perchlorate is that it gets stronger as it ages! You know how some cleaning agents and chemicals get weaker and less effective as they get older? Not this stuff. So, if you have an old bottle of bleach lying around, the amount of perchlorate will be much higher than in a newly manufactured bottle.[32]

Again, a small amount of this stuff soaking into your skin on occasion is probably no big deal for most of us. A sniff here and there? Probably okay. But daily or weekly exposures? We just don't know. And Ed and I have seen enough sick patients whose bodies were overburdened with these toxins that we suspect you're better off using something else.

The thing about many of the cleaners people like to use—especially in the era of COVID-19—is that they are super toxic. Yes, they kill germs, but if you read the label, most of them warn about eye irritants and against breathing in the vapors, and some even suggest you wear gloves while

32 *The Occurrence and Sources of Perchlorate in Massachusetts* (Boston: Massachusetts Department of Environmental Protection, 2005), www.waterboards.ca.gov/losangeles/water_issues/programs/remediation/perchlorate/05_0805_perchlorate-sources.pdf.

using them. Those are all signs you should not clean with them, at least not on a regular basis.

As you'll see in Chapter 9, there are coconut-based cleaners that will do the job of cleaning the bad germs for you, and vinegar will kill mold.

But this brings up another issue: not all bacteria are bad bacteria. And some of it is actually good for us. Honestly, it's better for your immune system if you are *not* pristine. In other words, don't scorch the earth simply to cut the grass.

One final note on cleaners—well, it's not really a cleaner, but it's kind of close. You know all those "air fresheners" people use? And those scented candles? If you have them, throw them away. Those fragrances are artificially created, usually with phthalates. You can use an orange-peel-derived spray to rid the bathroom of the stinky smell!

Keep in mind that this book is really focused on you and your home life. However, teachers aren't the only ones who work in toxic, mold-infested environments. Many of us are in just as much danger—if not more so—at work.

Are you a hairdresser who is dying hair or applying straighteners? Are you a nail salon person? Are you a painter or in construction?

What about being a plumber? Did you know that plumbers use some of the most toxic glues on the planet? And they use them on plastics! Glassblowers, factory workers—both can be extremely toxic positions. As can be anesthesiologists—they are exposed to all those gases they are pumping through to their patients. Oh, and did you know shipbuilders are at major risk? We had a patient who was a shipbuilder and was one of the most toxic people we've had in our practice. He had many of the common toxic symptoms and was losing his teeth too. And...and...and...

It's Scary!

We know all this can sound overwhelming. It may seem as if there are toxins everywhere (which there are) and that there's an enormous amount of work to do to protect yourself (which you might need to do). But take a deep breath and let your body relax for a second or two.

Now remind yourself that you didn't acquire a toxic life in the matter of a couple of weeks. It took years, maybe even decades, to get where you are.

So go easy with all this information. Read it and decide what *one thing* you can tackle now. After you tackle it, decide what *one thing* you can do next. And if you need help, see a Functional Medicine provider to get some.

A truly wonderful thing about the human body is that it does respond favorably to detoxification. It can heal and thrive, if given a chance. For some people, detoxification is relatively easy. Others have a hard time. It's all a matter of what's going on in their family tree.

Hot Top Tips

1. Inventory the potential toxins in your home and start systematically removing them.

   a. Cleaning supplies, soaps, and detergents

   b. Clothing

   c. Air fresheners

   d. Landscaping sprays and pesticides

   e. Tick and mosquito repellants

   f. Bleach

2. Evaluate where you feel best and worst and then have those areas tested for molds and air quality.

3. Visit the Environmental Working Group at www. ewg.org for lists of approved cleaners, skin products, and food.

CHAPTER 6

But Wait! You Really *Can* Blame Your Parents

Remember in Chapter 2 when we spoke about stress and methylation? We described how methylation is the body's method of getting toxins out of you. Well, some people are better methylators than others. It's a matter of genes. And I have sh*tty genes for methylating. After I looked at my genetic profile, I actually called my parents. "I'm delighted that you reproduced," I told them. "But, really, you never should have had children together."

My genes aren't the only things working against me, though. There are a couple of other things in the mix like my epigenetics, my lifestyle choices, and my response to stress.

Let's talk about genes first. Your genes influence everything from your hair and eye color to your risk of developing diabetes, heart disease, and, in my case, celiac disease. Having the gene determines whether you're at risk for any particular disease; it's not a guarantee that you'll get it. You need something to "turn on" a gene, and that brings us to epigenetics.

Epigenetics "is the study of how your behaviors and environment can cause changes that affect the way your genes work."[33] But epigenetics doesn't stop with just you; it includes the things your parents and grandparents experienced too. In my case, both my parents came from less-than-ideal backgrounds. They both had hard lives. My mom was born to struggling immigrants, and my father's parents and grandparents had pretty toxic relationships. While their issues may seem as if they have nothing to do with me, quite the opposite is true: my parents' and even my grandparents' life experiences impacted my DNA. That's what epigenetics is all about. And the same can be said for *your* parents' and grandparents' life experiences and *your* DNA.

So I was born to parents who each had their own issues, and their issues impacted me. As an infant, I had pneumonia, and as a child, I had repeated strep throat and ear infections. And as I grew up, I got antibiotics for *all* of them! This majorly messed up my microbiome. By the time I was in my teens and early twenties, I was well on my way to developing celiac (my genetic "overachievement" means I have not one gene, but *two* genes that put me at risk for celiac disease!). Unfortunately, celiac was poorly evaluated and diagnosed at that time, and gluten sensitivity was basically unheard of.

---

33 *"What Is Epigenetics?" Centers for Disease Control and Prevention, August 3, 2020,* www.cdc.gov/genomics/disease/epigenetics.htm.

Celiac disease is an autoimmune disease characterized by an allergy to gluten (gluten is a protein that is found in wheat and other grains), which then causes the lining of the gut to stop absorbing nutrients. Not surprisingly, I had malnutrition and iron deficiency that didn't respond to supplementation and persisted until I was diagnosed with celiac disease at age thirty-three! Untreated celiac patients are at risk for a ton of other issues, including osteoporosis, and are even more likely to die earlier!

Anytime a celiac eats gluten, the body mounts an immune attack. Specifically, the immune system attacks the person's small intestine, which leads to poor nutrient absorption. It can also cause a myriad of other health problems, such as brain fog, asthma, joint pain, weight gain/loss, hypertension, fatigue, and more. You can have sensitivity to gluten without having celiac disease or even the genes for celiac, but you must have the genes in order to develop celiac. And you don't need two genes to develop celiac; you can develop it with only one.

I, however, got *two* genes and, as a result of my parents' issues, likely got genes that were more apt to cause celiac. (By the way, did I mention that my father and one of my brothers have celiac? That my first cousins have gluten sensitivity? And that my mother has had multiple autoimmune diseases? Yep, terrible genes!) So I suffered malnutrition that was never able to be righted with supplements.

Having celiac caused other problems for me, too, like asthma, low thyroid function, thinning hair, brain fog, infertility (made up for that one!), and irritable bowel syndrome, which, again, wasn't something that was diagnosed and treated until I was an adult. (Instead, I grew up thinking everybody just had a better cork than I did.)

Celiac made me more susceptible to multiple food sensitivities that subsequently impacted my health in ways that just weren't recognized when I was growing up. Something the medical community knows now but didn't back then is that food allergies and intolerances do more than cause tummy troubles. They can easily result in poor concentration, irritability, drama fits, and even anxiety and depression. So considering my undiagnosed celiac, it's easy to see why I might have sometimes been a little bitchy, which my mother will confirm!

Then, when you top that life cocktail with a type-A personality that runs fast, hard, and gives everything she's got, a lot of stress is the result. I didn't just get my master's in business administration *or* go to medical school—I did a combination of both at the same time. I didn't do a residency at a quiet suburban hospital; I moved to the Bronx in New York City, where I worked eighty-hour weeks. Then I had four kids! Stress was just part and parcel of my life...until I learned better.

But there's nothing like illness to teach you a lesson.

Not everyone has celiac, so I realize my particular situation is a little more complicated compared to many. The point I'm trying to make here is that people who are genetically predisposed to particular illnesses often also have a more difficult time detoxing. Celiac is just one such illness. However, just because you might be predisposed to something doesn't mean it will manifest in your body—that's where your epigenetics comes into play. They are the switch that turns a gene on or off. Regardless, it's always a good idea to see what you may be predisposed to, which is why we recommend many of our patients get a DNA test.

Knockoff and Designer Genes

When we order a DNA test for a patient, we're looking for a number of things. First, we want to see if that person is genetically predisposed to gluten sensitivities or other food-related issues. Second, we look for genes that could influence the way the patient processes nutrients and detoxes. In particular, we look at genes that govern:

- Lipid metabolism

- Methylation

- Detoxification

- Inflammation

- Oxidative stress

- Bone health

- Insulin sensitivity

- Iron overload

- Caffeine sensitivity

- Salt sensitivity

What we try to do with the information we get from your DNA profile is put together a picture that tells us what your risk is for developing something based on your genes. That doesn't take into account your lifestyle or epigenetics. But it does allow us to look backward and compare what's going on in your genes with what's going on in your health now. If you have bad toxic issues and we look at your genes, it's possible we can say, "Of course you're having problems! This is why." And that allows us to put together a protocol that takes into consideration what your genes are trying to do.

For example, one of the key genes we look at is the MTHFR. I have a specific name for it—if you put a potty mouth on your imagination, you can probably guess what it is. And if you need another hint, let's look at it like this: if you inherit a mutation in that gene from both your parents, then you're ~insert word for screwed here~ when it comes to methylation.

Guess what? I have two mutated MTHFR genes. That's one of the many reasons I'm such a crappy methylator and became such a hot toxic mess. Here's a snapshot of my profile:

GENE AND VARIATION	RSID[34]	ALLELES	RESULT
COMT V158M	rs4680	AG	+ / −
COMT H62H	rs4633	CT	+ / −
COMT P199P	rs769224	GG	− / −
VDR Bsm	rs1544410	CT	+ / −
VDR Taq	rs731236	AG	+ / −
MTHFR C677T	rs1801133	AA	+ / +

---

34 The rsID number is a unique label ("rs" followed by a number) used by researchers and databases to identify a specific SNP (Single Nucleotide Polymorphism). It stands for Reference SNP cluster ID and is the naming convention used for most SNPs.

GENE AND VARIATION	RSID[35]	ALLELES	RESULT
MTHFR A1298C	rs1801131	TT	– / –
MTR A2756G	rs1805087	AA	– / –
MTRR A66G	rs1801394	AG	+ / –
MTRR K350A	rs162036	AA	– / –
MTRR R415T	rs2287780	CC	– / –
BHMT-02	rs567754	CC	– / –
CBS C699T	rs234706	GG	– / –
SHMT1 C1420T	rs1979277	AG	+ / –

We spoke about methylation in Chapter 2 when we discussed stress. But, because it can be a complicated topic, here is a quick rundown: methylation happens when a small molecule (called a methyl group) is added to other molecules. That might sound innocent, as if it's just a harmless attempt to be with the popular kids. After all, the human body has so many molecules that to say it as a number it would be seven billion billion billion. But, although tiny, those molecules add up like those pounds around my midsection before I discovered my toxic body burden. In fact, they *did* add up to those pounds around my midsection. Because here's the thing: if you don't properly methylate, you can't properly synthesize the vitamins and minerals to nourish your body. That includes the precious methyl groups donated by your B vitamins that are required for binding and eliminating toxins.

---

35   The rsID number is a unique label ("rs" followed by a number) used by researchers and databases to identify a specific SNP (Single Nucleotide Polymorphism). It stands for Reference SNP cluster ID and is the naming convention used for most SNPs.

That's a key point to remember here: proper methylation is needed for detoxing.

If both your parents gave you a normal MTHFR gene (along with other genes), your body will be able to convert folate and vitamin B12 into their active forms—"active forms" means they get a "methyl" group added onto them, which then gives your body a source for donation/binding/excretion. In other words, they enable you to poop out toxins. For folks like me, who have two mutated MTHFR genes, our ability to make that conversion happen is impaired by 60 to 90 percent. So, since we cannot methylate those B vitamins, we have a hard time using their methyl groups for binding and eliminating toxins.

The consequences of having mutated MTHFR genes extend beyond detoxification. When MTHFR genes are mutated, they can't help the vitamins and nutrients turn into the forms they need to be in, in order for you to maintain good health (or even survive). To show you what I mean, let's look at homocysteine.

Homocysteine levels can be checked with regular lab work. And the reason a doctor would order that test is because elevated homocysteine levels are a risk factor for cardiovascular disease, heart attack, and stroke. But that's not all. Homocysteine is a nonessential, sulfur-containing, non-proteinogenic amino acid. In order for it to make proteins, it needs activated vitamins B12, B6, and folic acid.[36] So if those are not methylated (activated) due to the mutated MTHFR genes, they can't do their job of changing homocysteine into the protein your body needs to excrete. Then what happens is that you have an abundance of homocysteine floating around in your body, which, again, puts you at risk for heart disease and strokes. So if we see someone with MTHFR genes *and* high homocysteine levels, then we may try a specific protocol of activated vitamin B supplementation to help their body achieve lower levels of homocysteine and therefore lower their risk for heart disease.

The good news is that by knowing what's at work in your DNA, we can create specific supplemental protocols to help you (and me) get the vitamin Bs and all the other nutrients we need for detoxification and overall health.

While a person's genetics do help Ed and me create treatment protocols custom-tailored to their DNA and unique needs, we know their genes are only part of the picture. And we also know our genes don't call all the shots. Just because you have a gene for something doesn't mean it will manifest in your life. Like, sure, I have crappy genetics for celiac disease, but if I had been

---

36 Henrieta Škovierová et al., "The Molecular and Cellular Effect of Homocysteine Metabolism Imbalance on Human Health," International Journal of Molecular Sciences 17, no. 10 (2016): 1733, www.ncbi.nlm.nih.gov/pmc/articles/ PMC5085763/#:~:text=Homocysteine%20(Hcy)%20is%20a%20non,Hcy%20 is%20produced%20in%20humans.

born into an ideal world and had had a stress- and trouble-free life, those genes may never have expressed themselves, in which case I could eat as many soft pretzels as I wanted.

Likewise, there are people with genes for Parkinson's, Alzheimer's, and even breast cancer who will never develop those diseases because nothing made their genes express themselves. But few—if any—people actually grow up in an ideal world where such triggers never happen. Instead, a person's epigenetics can come into play and pull some triggers.

Epi Who?

So your DNA is your book of life. It's immutable; it doesn't change. However, it's not the kind of book that you read from beginning to end. You can pop in and out of that story at any point, and what makes you do that popping about is governed by your epigenetics—the things that happen to you, or that happened to your parents and even your grandparents, that subsequently influence your genes.

Epigenetics includes our current environment, our past, what was happening with our mother when we were in her womb, our father around the time we were conceived, what both parents' lives were like when they were going through puberty, and even how healthy our grandparents were. For example, studies in Sweden have shown that when a man experiences a famine while going through puberty, his grandchildren are statistically and significantly less likely to experience heart disease, cancer, and diabetes! In contrast, the grandchildren of men who had a feast period of their life during puberty are significantly more likely to experience heart disease, cancer, diabetes, and earlier death.[37]

So when we talk to patients, we need to look at what's going on in their bodies DNA-wise as well as what happened in their life history to see what we're working with or against in order to get them healthy. In my case, my dad was ill when I was conceived and shortly after I was born. As I mentioned, my mom's family were immigrants who had numerous financial and health stressors, and my mom was deeply impacted by those issues. It was a toxic environment for her in that sense, so it's reasonable to assume that her stress load impacted the way my DNA was read when I was in the womb and even when I was a child living in that environment.

An experiment done on mice is probably one of the best examples of just how powerful an influence epigenetics can be. In 2000, researchers at Duke University wanted to see if they could impact the genes in agouti mice; their name comes from the fact that they carry a gene called the agouti gene. What's so special about that gene is that it makes mice fat and yellow—it also makes them prone to diabetes and cancer.

---

37   Denny Vågerö et al., "Paternal Grandfather's Access to Food Predicts All-Cause and Cancer Mortality in Grandsons," *Nature Communications* 9 (2018), www.nature.com/articles/s41467-018-07617-9.

Typically, when an agouti male mates with an agouti female, they produce genetically identical agouti offspring: fat, yellow mice who usually die from diabetes or cancer. That's what their genes "dictate" them to be and do. However, for the experiment, the team at Duke fed the moms a diet rich in B vitamins, including folate, and other nutrients that contained methyl groups.

The results? The agouti gene did not "turn on." The babies were born slender...and brown! But they were still genetically identical to their mom and dad![38]

For young people growing up in an environment that is perpetually stressful, when they are in a constant state of fight-flight-or-freeze, their worst epigenetic-influenced traits come out. Layer on a standard American diet (SAD) that is devoid of fresh vegetables, too much screen time, and too little physical exercise, and the body leans toward inflammation, which compounds as they get older.

As with my celiac genes, there are a lot of people who have predispositions to various diseases. However, they may never get those diseases unless they go through a stressful period, or suffer trauma, or eat the wrong foods for too long, or get exposed to too many toxins, or all of the above.

---

38 "Environmental Influence," Stanford at the Tech Understanding Genetics, April 7, 2011, https://genetics.thetech.org/ask/ask403#:~:text=Sometimes%20a%20 brown%20mouse%20has,and%20toxins%20from%20around%20us.

Yes, I'm aware that this might sound scary or even depressing. DNA and epigenetics are things that are totally out of our control. So I get it: you might be freaking out right now because you grew up in a dysfunctional family three blocks away from a nuclear power plant. But I promise you, there is hope! All is not lost!

Hope

A really good thing about DNA is that it tells you what you *can* do to improve your life. Do you have a gene that says you're predisposed to celiac? Then stay away from gluten—not just in the form of eating it; look for personal care products that say they are gluten-free, and don't work in a bakery. If your DNA suggests you might be prone to high cholesterol, then there are things that you can eat and exercise strategies that you can do that will counter the DNA.

Are you curious about how your family history could be impacting your health? You can get DNA tests done through labs like Ancestry or 23andMe. Then, when you get your results, have a Functional Medicine doctor help you figure out what they might mean for you.

Regardless of what your genes may say, what's most important to remember is that by attending to the fundamentals of good health, you can circumnavigate many—if not all—of the woes your DNA may want to wreak on you. That means you get enough quality sleep to let your body recover every night. It means you eat the right foods to ensure proper nutrition and proper elimination. It means you surround yourself with healthy relationships and release the toxic ones. And it means you move your body on a regular basis. You don't have to run marathons or become a Ms. Universe bodybuilder contestant. But you do want to give your body the movement it wants and needs to stay strong, supple, and able.

Always remember, your DNA is just a list of ingredients for you to make a life soup with. How that soup turns out is a matter of what you do with those ingredients. And you know what? It's never too late to change the recipe. In fact, science is beginning to suggest that there is no tipping point, that no matter what, you can become healthier and healthier as you age and reverse the problems plaguing you—even the ones you have a genetic predisposition toward.

Don't believe me? It sounds crazy, but Harvard Medical School professor David Sinclair and a team of researchers were able to reverse aging in mice. They used a technique called partial cellular reprogramming, which reset epigenetic alterations in the cells of mice that had caused age-related blindness. Yes, they were able to make the blind mice see again![39]

In addition to the groundbreaking work Dr. Sinclair is doing, people like Terry Wahls, a Functional Medicine doctor who was

---

39   Steve Hill et al., "Reversing Age-Related Vision Loss Using Cellular Reprogram-ming," Lifespan.io, August 6, 2019, https://www.lifespan.io/news/reversing-age-re-lated-vision-loss-using-cellular-reprogramming/.

once wheelchair-bound, are spreading a similar word: you *can* reverse disease! She was in an advanced stage of the autoimmune disease multiple sclerosis. Once confined to a wheelchair, she is now walking around on stages giving talks about how she healed herself mostly by changing her diet! How cool is that?

However, before you can reverse any damage, you need to know what that damage looks like now. How dirty are you?

Hot Top Tips

1. If possible, get a clear family history so you can look for trends.

2. Get your genetic test done through Ancestry, 23andMe, or another DNA service.

3. Run that data through an interpretive program to see what your methylation, detox, and other genes put you at risk for.

4. Guard your weak side! Get a consult from a Functional Medicine provider to optimize your health!

5. Give your body what it needs: get enough sleep, minimize processed foods, and move your body regularly. And Manage. Your. Stress!

CHAPTER 7

Diagnosis: You're Dirty

I wanted to rip my face off. I was that miserable. It started as a runny nose. Since it was February, I assumed my constant drip had something to do with an early allergy season kicking in since it was already so warm. But it got worse. My nose just wouldn't stop running, and then the skin around it and above my lip became red and itchy. I knew it wasn't from me blowing my nose. I was careful and used a safe cream to tend to it. But then the rash wouldn't go away either. It also didn't respond to antifungal cream or topical steroid cream.

Instead, the rash grew and expanded until it covered the sides of my nose and spread out from my nostrils by about a centimeter. Meanwhile, the drip continued. It's a good thing I had already been married for several years; otherwise, I'd have had a problem trying to date!

Things only worsened. The rash went from being red, unsightly, and itchy to being red, unsightly, and burning as it continued to grow! It then appeared on my chin and eyelids! My whole face itched so badly that, yes, I seriously wanted to rip my face off. What the hell could be causing it?

I had been detoxing from mold, which usually makes rashes go away—not do the opposite. The only thing Ed and I could think of was that the rash was candida, a yeast overgrowth. Yeast is usually a sign of too much sugar consumption. But since my diet happened to be pretty d*mned good during this period of my life, I knew it was something else. I suspected heavy metals, as yeast often shows up when an excess of them are floating around in your body. And heavy metals kind of made sense. I had tested myself a few months previously and found lead levels that were a few points above the upper limit of normal and borderline high mercury. So I had followed through with a protocol to remove them. I then felt so good that I figured the metals were gone and had yet to get around to doing the post-treatment test that would check to see if any were still present.

But let's back up a second: why did we think it was yeast? Well, yeast *thrives* when there is a lot of sugar in the body or when the immune system is suppressed, especially by metals. So now you might be wondering why I didn't have a yeast overgrowth on my skin when I had tested positive for metals in the first place. That's because before detoxing, the metals were, for the most part, hiding in my fat and not circulating in my bloodstream. We believe the yeast flared so much at that time because I had started the metals detox, which brought them out of storage so I could eliminate them. But then, thinking the metals were gone, I had stopped the detox, leaving the metals with easy access to suppress the immune system and make me more susceptible to yeast overgrowth.

Regardless, it was clear I needed to up my detox game to get this stuff out of me! So I finally got around to doing my metals retest and, yep, it was positive. Only this time, it wasn't *slightly* out of range. The results were much higher. On one hand, this was discouraging, since I was much farther away from being "done" than I had thought. On the other hand, this was good news. As we'll explain later, because we test for toxins by measuring what you are eliminating, we have no way of quantifying what is in your body. So what happens is that as you start the detox process, it's like turning on a rusted spigot: at first a trickle of toxins are pulled out to be eliminated, but as you continue to detox, it's as if you crank that spigot all the way open and the toxins come out in larger amounts. When I did my first round of testing, it was at a time when my body had essentially been locked down. It wasn't able to rid itself of the toxins. The first round of detox "woke it up." So I promptly started another round of the metals removal protocol and added in alpha-lipoic acid, which helps your body create glutathione, which is what your liver needs to bind the toxins.

Guess what? My rash resolved itself within forty-eight hours.

Skin issues are probably the most common signs of a toxic body. But they are not the only sign. Here is a questionnaire to see if you may be exhibiting signs of toxicity.

Use the following scale to rate each of the listed symptoms based on how they have impacted your health and well-being over the past thirty days:[40]

---

40   This set questionnaire is based on the Medical Symptom Questionnaire from the Institute of Functional Medicine.

0 = Never, or almost never, experienced the symptom

1 = Occasionally experienced it, but it is not severe

2 = Occasionally experienced it, and it is severe

3 = Frequently experienced it, but it is not severe

4 = Frequently experienced it, and it is severe

DIGESTIVE TRACT	
Nausea or vomiting	
Diarrhea	
Constipation	
Bloating	
Belching, passing gas	
Heartburn/indigestion	
Stomach or intestinal pain	
Total	

EARS	
Itchy ears	
Earaches or infections	
Drainage	
Ringing, tinnitus, or hearing loss	
Total	

EMOTIONS	
Mood swings	
Anxiety, panic attacks, nervousness	
Anger, irritability, aggression	
Depression	
Total	

ENERGY	
Fatigue or feeling sluggish	
Apathy, lethargy	
Hyperactivity	
Restlessness	
Total	

EYES	
Itchy and/or watery	
Swollen, red, and/or sticky/gooey eyelids	
"Bags"—dark circles under eyes	
Blurred or tunnel vision	
Total	

HEAD/SLEEP	
Headaches	
Faintness	
Dizziness	
Insomnia	
Total	

HEART	
Irregular or skipped beating	
Rapid or pounding beating	
Chest pain	
Total	

JOINTS AND MUSCLES	
Joint pain or aches	
Arthritis	
Stiffness, limited movement	
Muscle aches or pain	
Feeling physically week or tired	
Total	

LUNGS	
Chest congestion/mucus	
Asthma or bronchitis	
Shortness of breath	
Difficulty breathing	
Total	

MIND	
Poor memory	
Confusion / poor comprehension	
Poor concentration	
Poor physical coordination	
Difficulty in making decisions	
Stuttering or stammering	
Slurred speech	
Learning disabilities	
Total	

MOUTH AND THROAT	
Chronic coughing	
Gagging or frequently clearing throat	
Sore throat, hoarseness, or loss of voice	
Swollen/discolored tongue, gums, lips	
Canker sores	
Total	

NOSE	
Stuffiness	
Sinus problems	
Hay fever	
Sneezing attacks	
Excessive mucus	
Total	

SKIN	
Acne	
Hives, rashes, or dry skin	
Hair loss	
Flushing or hot flushes	
Excessive sweating	
Total	

WEIGHT	
Binge eating or drinking	
Cravings	
Excessive weight	
Compulsive eating	

Water retention	
Underweight	
Total	

OTHER	
Frequently ill	
Frequent need for or urgent urination	
Genital itch or discharge	
Total	

Now add all your totals for a grand total: _____

To determine your potential toxicity level, use this scale:

Less than 10 = Optimal health (congratulations!)

Between 10 and 50 = Suggests mild toxicity

Between 50 and 100 = Suggests moderate toxicity

Over 100 = Suggests severe toxicity

Getting Professional Help

Now, if you're still reading this, that probably means you think you might be a dirty girl (or guy) after all. If so, and you want to get clean, then you might be tempted to reach out to your primary care doctor. But that might not be the best approach for you. Not all doctors will have knowledge of or training in this approach. Your primary care doctor is a well-educated and well-trained physician. Primary care doctors are trained to diagnose conditions and treat them with medications. They're very useful and needed for your overall health. Ed is also a primary care doctor.

However, just as you sometimes need to go to a gastroenterologist for specific problems related to your stomach or digestive system, or a pulmonologist for lung-related problems, there are times when you need to go to a Functional Medicine doctor. Gastro docs and pulmonologists each get years of additional training in their respective fields outside of their primary care education. Similarly, Functional Medicine doctors get years of additional training. In particular, Functional Medicine doctors get extra training in the fundamentals of the biochemical processes of the body and how to impact them through optimizing nutrition and lifestyle, and mitigating the influence of stress, toxins, and genetics. Although Ed still sees some patients as a primary care doctor, and I still see some gynecological patients, we have almost two decades of post-residency training and experience in the specialty field of Functional Medicine.

Functional Medicine doctors are trained to find the root cause—or causes—of illness. We look for what could be triggering it or exacerbating symptoms and work to eliminate or manage those triggers as best as possible.

We hope you have a robust and trusting relationship with your primary care doctor, and we encourage you to continue that relationship. However, you will want to find a Functional Medicine practice, like Five Journeys, the one Ed and I run, to discuss whether your health concerns could be related to toxins and get to the root cause of your illness.

You can find an experienced Functional Medicine doctor on the Institute for Functional Medicine's website, www.ifm. org. While Functional Medicine doctors aren't as common as primary care physicians, many, like us, offer telemedicine appointments. There are no bounds to our practice in the United States. And most of the lab work we recommend can be done either in your home or at the same local lab your primary care doctor sends you to.

Even though we often use the same labs as your primary care doctor, we differ in what we're looking for. Typically, Functional Medicine tests are more extensive in nature and set a higher standard for desired results. We look at and interpret the testing differently. Because we're not just going for average results so you can scrape by feeling "all right," we don't just do *average* testing on you and look for *average* results. We have stricter requirements. Take B12, for example. Conventional doctors will tell you an acceptable low level of B12 is between 300 and 350. We prefer to see that number at 800 or above. And when conventional docs look at your hemoglobin A1C, which measures your average blood sugar over the previous three months, they diagnose you as diabetic if that number is above 6.4 and prediabetic if it's between 5.7 and 6.4, though many physicians prefer a number below 6.5, and some push a little harder and like the numbers below 5.7. Our criteria are even stricter; we like people's A1C at least below 5.7 but work hard to get them under 5.4.

Those are just a few places where we differ from conventional lab expectations. There are many, many more—too many to discuss here. And, really, there is so much more for you to know about the functional approach to medicine and your health.

A Functional Approach

While getting to the root cause of your illness is a main concern for Functional Medicine doctors, it's not our only concern for our patients. For our patients, we don't think just alleviating their symptoms is enough. Our aim is for them to achieve optimum levels of health. **Ed and I honestly believe you are meant to feel freaking amazing until you are at least one hundred years old.**

We believe the body *wants* to be well. So when you are symptomatic, that tells us either your body doesn't have enough of something (hormones, nutrients, etc.) or that it has too much of something (food allergies, gut issues/imbalances, environmental toxins, heavy metals, pesticides, mycotoxins, etc.). Our approach adds back in what your body needs and gets rid of what it doesn't by using both conventional and specialty testing to determine what's high and what's low. When we do that, your body can heal itself.

Even if we assume someone's health issues are related to toxins, we don't automatically check for them as the first step with our patients. For most patients, we first need to make sure you have a healthy platform, a decent framework in place before we even *start* talking about toxins. That means we make sure that you have a healthy gut and that your hormones and micronutrients are balanced. We want to make sure you're eating well and sleeping well, and we want to know about the stressors in your life.

While that all might sound like a lot (because it is), Ed and I have a systematic approach to cover all our bases. Often, we will evaluate your gut health, which we typically do through a stool test. Testing your stool can tell us whether you've got a problem with your microbiome: an imbalance, a yeast overgrowth, impaired digestion, or a flat-out infection. If any of those issues are present, they will need to be fixed before any kind of detoxing will be successful.

Micro Who?

Your gut is not one solid, stretchy layer of tissue. Instead, the approximately two thousand square feet of surface that makes up your intestinal lining is populated by a wide range of bacteria (good and bad), viruses, fungi, and other living organisms, which, combined, is called your microbiome. All the stuff that comes into your gut—all the foods you eat, in what combination, along with the (mostly unavoidable) toxins—impacts the microbiome to either make it stronger or weaker.

Fun fact: the microbiome of an average adult weighs around five pounds.[41]

41 Erin P. Ferranti et al., "20 Things You Didn't Know about the Human Gut Microbiome," *The Journal of Cardiovascular Nursing* 29, no. 6 (2014): 479–481, www.ncbi. nlm.nih.gov/pmc/articles/PMC4191858

Clean, nutritious food supports a strong and healthy microbiome. On the other hand, there are so many other things that can impact it in an unhealthy way. Toxins such as pesticides, lead, and plastic disrupt it. Many medicines, like NSAIDs (nonsteroidal anti-inflammatories like Motrin or Aleve) and steroids can damage it. In particular, the rampant use of proton pump inhibitors such as Prilosec has become a real concern because of its negative impact on the microbiome. And interestingly, but perhaps not surprisingly, when you think about the impact of stress, even our thoughts can impact our microbiome.

You might be wondering what the big deal is. After all, if the microbiome is just a bunch of bacteria and fungi (ew!), then why worry about it? Well, here's why: your microbiome plays an important role in just about everything!

- Mood and emotions
- Immune system
- Digestion
- Aging
- Nutrient balance
- Autoimmunity
- Weight
- Blood sugar control
- Hormones
- And on and on

In short, your microbiome is where your emotional and physical health originates. And, yes, you read that sentence correctly: your microbiome is where your *emotional* and physical health originates.

Let's look at the emotional side first. Our microbiome is where many of our neurotransmitters and hormones call home, and they communicate with you through your emotions. Have you ever had a gut feeling? Something inside you telling you that something isn't quite right? Or, opposite that, have you ever felt your intuition saying that something is definitely right? That's your microbiome at work. It's often called the second brain because it has so many neurotransmitters in it. Additionally, several hormones are produced in our microbiome that affect our moods. In particular, about 80 percent of our serotonin production happens there. Serotonin is our happy hormone; it promotes feelings of well-being, positivity, and joy. There are studies that show a correlation between gut health and serotonin modulation, suggesting that if your gut is impaired in some way (including by toxins), your serotonin levels can fluctuate.[42] And a key factor in making folks prone to depression and anxiety is impaired serotonin function. In short, a healthy gut helps you stay happy![43]

And on the physical health side, your microbiome houses about 70 percent of the cells that make up your immune

---

42 Cristina Stasi, Sinan Sadalla, and Stefano Milani, "The Relationship between the Serotonin Metabolism, Gut-Microbiota and the Gut-Brain Axis," *Current Drug Metabolism* 20, no. 8 (2019): 646–655, https://pubmed.ncbi.nlm.nih.gov/31345143/.

43 Philip J. Cowen and Michael Browning, "What Has Serotonin to Do with Depression?" *World Psychiatry* 14, no. 2 (2015): 158–160, https://www.ncbi.nlm.nih.gov/pmc/articles/PMC4471964/.

system. These cells require healthy bacteria to thrive—the "good" bacteria you may have heard of in TV commercials about yogurt.

We can't talk about yogurt without bringing up sugar. It's troubling that so many yogurts are sold as "healthy" foods, when they're loaded with sugar. We usually don't recommend much cow dairy in general, and if it's filled with sugar that just erases all the positives you could get from the probiotics in the yogurt. We recommend unsweetened goat's yogurt or unsweetened dairy alternatives like coconut, soy, or almond yogurts.

The microbiome also plays an important role when it comes to detoxing. One of its primary jobs is to break down and digest food into vitamins and minerals. Part of that includes methylating your B vitamins, which are necessary for detoxing. In other words, if your microbiome isn't functioning optimally, your body will not function at its best because it won't be able to detox properly.

When we talk about your gut functioning optimally or not, we're often talking about something called increased intestinal permeability, or leaky gut.

When Your Gut Leaks

The cells that line your gut are fused together; their membranes, or cell walls, kind of smash up against each other in what we call "tight junctions." While those cells seem to be stuck together as if they are glued, the tight junctions can loosen and even open up. Should they open frequently or stay open for long periods, a condition called leaky gut can develop. That's when larger particles of any bacteria, food, or toxins you may have ingested now have an opportunity to pass directly into your bloodstream instead of getting eliminated.

Prednisone, NSAIDs, alcohol, trauma, steroids, food sensitivities, and poor nutrition all raise the chance of developing leaky gut. Stress, with that whole slowing-digestion bit, can also aid in the development of leaky gut. As can highly processed foods, sugar, and gluten.

NSAIDs are nonsteroidal anti-inflammatory drugs that are commonly taken for pain relief. They include ibuprofen, high-dose aspirin, naproxen, celecoxib, mefenamic acid, etoricoxib, and indomethacin. Some of those words may be unfamiliar, but the next time you have a headache or are feeling some joint pain and reach for something to alleviate it (yep, Aleve is an NSAID too), read the ingredients. You may be surprised to find one of these listed.

Gluten? As in wheat? Gluten can cause gut problems? Yep. Gluten, a protein found in wheat, barley, rye, malt, and several other grains, can make the junctions open up for about fifteen minutes before closing again. However, if you are someone who is genetically sensitive to wheat gluten (meaning you're not only sensitive to eating gluten, but you also carry the genetic risk for celiac disease), those tight junctions in your gut lining open for about four hours after eating wheat.

> To have a genetic predisposition for gluten sensitivity, that means you carry DQ2 or DQ8 genetic mutations on the HLA subtypes. It is estimated that up to 40 percent of the population has one or even both of those gene mutations. But just because you have the gene mutation doesn't mean you'll develop a sensitivity or even celiac. There have to be other triggers. And both stress and overexposure to toxins can be prime triggers.

Now do the math with those numbers—either fifteen minutes or four hours, it doesn't really matter—and think about how often people eat gluten. They have bagels, toast, or danishes with breakfast and wraps, burgers, or sandwiches for lunch. Pretzels or crackers for a midafternoon snack? Then what's for dinner? There's often some kind of bread, even when there's pasta on the plate. And look at our favorite desserts: cakes, pies, pastries,

and cookies! If you carry one or both of the genes, exposure to
gluten that frequently can cause you to have nearly constant
communication between your intestines and your bloodstream.
And therein lies the danger. Have mycotoxins, environmental
toxins, pesticides, preservatives, artificial colors and flavors, or
bacteria in your gut? Oh, yep, then they're in your bloodstream,
too, as are larger particles of food.

So now your blood is cruising along, doing its thing, spreading oxygen and red blood cells and nutrients everywhere
they need to go, when it meets up with the substances
coming through your leaky gut. In comes some weird sh*t,
some bacteria and chemicals that are not supposed to be in
your body.

"What the hell is this?" your blood wants to know. But there is
no one around who can answer. So, a little confused, it decides
the best course of action is twofold. One: it will mount an
immune response to fight off the bacteria and attack the food
particles. And two: it will sequester the toxins away in some fat,
bones, or organs until a better answer comes along. The first
response results in your body developing antibodies against the
food particles it's seeing and also means you gain weight that's
loaded with toxins.

Then what ends up happening is that people come in to see
Ed and me, suffering from rashes, headaches, nonexistent
libido, or constant fatigue—things that happen when your
immune system is doing its job against an assailant. But a few
other things happen when your body mounts that immune

attack. You can start developing food sensitivities, which is bad enough. But, something much worse, you can develop an auto-immune disease.

On the molecular level, food particles often look like something that isn't supposed to be in your body. So when your body comes across these particles, it creates an immune response to attack that food. This overactivation can also cause other inappropriate immune activation, leading to other autoimmune diseases or inflammatory diseases like cancer, heart disease, Alzheimer's, Hashimoto's, type 1 diabetes, Crohn's, ulcerative colitis, celiac, rheumatoid arthritis, psoriasis, and eczema, among others.

Leaky gut can also contribute to women having menstrual abnormalities and to almost everyone having some kind of tummy troubles, whether that's bloating and gas, constipation, or diarrhea. Weight gain, weight loss, and nutritional deficiencies are rampant too. And all of those may be signs and symptoms of a leaky gut. It can get so extreme, the immune response can get so amped up, that your body starts reacting to everything as if it's an enemy. Then nothing you eat will sit well with you. We've had patients tell us their gut is so out of whack that they feel like they react to air and water!

But when you have a healthy balance of bacteria in your microbiome and normal stomach acid (which we'll discuss in the next chapter), then your methylation happens and your bloodstream is not given an opportunity to throw a big dramatic fit with your immune system.

We did an experiment in our office in 2013. We bought a hamburger from McDonald's and another from Burger King and let them sit out in our office, on display in a plastic box.

They are still sitting in our front office, looking almost identical to the day we bought them. No mold, no fungus; nothing is growing on them. The bread is just stale.

What that means is that bacteria won't eat the burgers. In which case, we have to ask, how can we tell if this is food? And if bacteria won't eat it, how can you expect your body to digest it?

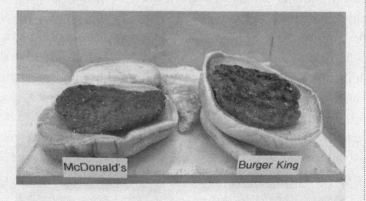

In other words, fast food is often not truly food. Which explains why obese people who frequently eat it are actually malnourished. The "foods" are calorie-dense, but nutrient-poor.

So now you know why gut health is important in general. But the primary reason we bring it up in this book is because of that whole methylation factor. If you're going to go through a detox protocol, you need to be able to properly methylate the toxins (remember, that means that your body binds them so you can eliminate them). And to properly methylate, you need a healthy gut.

Gut dysfunction can make it difficult to detox, since the digestive system is focused on more pressing issues that are required for survival. Detox is a "thrive" behavior, and gut function is necessary for survival. So we have to normalize the gut first before we tackle higher-order needs such as detoxification.

But that's not all that's required to get your body in the right state before detoxing. There is more that Ed and I will look at.

Prepping the Rest of Your Platform

As you now know, DNA is a key element to your health. So, as part of your workup with us, you may need to collect spit samples so we can check your DNA for your genetic risk for disease. We'll also use spit samples to run tests on your cortisol levels in order to help us get an idea about how well your adrenals are functioning.

As part of your basic blood lab work, we'll check for possible food sensitivities and examine your nutritional levels. We'll look for both deficiencies and overages, and we may look at your micronutrient status, too, which is done with both blood work and urine lab tests. We also look for evidence of significant infections that can throw off your health, like Lyme disease or Epstein-Barr.

Outside of all the lab work and the data that gives us, we want information that only talking to you will provide. So we will take our time to get to know you.

Getting to Know You

Functional Medicine docs want to know more than just what's going on in your body chemistry. We're going to ask so many questions, you might start wondering if you're on a hidden-camera dating game show. We'll want to know all about your lifestyle. How well do you sleep? How stressed are you on a regular basis? Got a sex drive? If not, are you still able to orgasm? What is your relationship like with your family, your peers, and yourself? We may not ask everyone every question, but we are pretty nosy and want to understand your life and your history.

We'll want to know what you do to take care of yourself. This involves the kind of exercise or body movement you really get on a regular basis, your diet, and how you manage stress.

Your relationships will be important to us, including friendships, work relationships, family relationships, and love relationships. Yes, we may want to know how things are in bed because, seriously, if the answer is "not great," then that needs to be addressed!

We'll want the full history of you, and not just to get an idea of what kind of health problems you had in the past, but we'll want to know what could have affected your epigenetics. So we may ask about your childhood and what your family life was like as you grew up. Similarly, what was school life like for you? Whether you were social with healthy, happy peers or you struggled with academics or with fitting in can really impact your health as an adult. Everyone has had some kind of trauma in their life; have you peeled back the layers on yours?

Because food is so important, we'll want to know what your relationship with food is and has been like for you. We'll also probably discuss your eating habits to determine if, or how much, you've consumed fast food and how prevalent plastics were in your life in connection with food. We may even ask you to define what you think a healthy diet is now and to describe what you eat on a regular basis now.

And we'll be so nosy, we might ask about how satisfied you are with your job or whether you have hobbies.

By the time we're done asking questions, you might want to double-check whether you went to the right office; perhaps you stumbled into a therapist's practice by mistake. But have no worries; we won't forget why you came to visit us.

At this point, we'll know where you stand regarding gut health, nutrient and hormone balance, and adrenal health. We can then work on bringing you up to optimum health in those areas. But if you are in a good enough place—or once you get there—and we still suspect toxins, we can now test for them.

Why the wait? Well, after getting the basic testing done, if we feel there are major issues at that point, that's what we'll address first. Those changes usually fall in the realm of diet and lifestyle changes. Once we think you're healthy enough, if you're still showing symptoms of toxicity, then we'll order toxin labs. Of course, for every rule, there is an exception. There have been a few patients we've seen who were so sick, we started with toxins. But they are the exceptions, not the rule.

We do it in that order because detoxing can be stressful on the body, so you want to be as bolstered up as possible before you start. And those labs will also help us know how well your body is detoxing on its own already. Remember that whole methylation thing? Well, when we mentioned we do a nutritional analysis through your lab work, that includes running labs to look for vitamins B12, folate levels, and homocysteine levels. If those are off, that can indicate that you don't have the substrates necessary to process toxins properly, so we'll need to help your body first by supplementing those nutrients.

Once you're ready, we can look at toxins.

Am I Toxic?

Remember when we mentioned that your bloodstream recognizes that toxins are bad for you, so it quickly gets them to a storage place (fat, bones, and tissues)? Because of that, toxins rarely show up in blood lab results. If they are there, that means you may have had a very recent exposure and the toxin is on its way to storage. Or, worse, it means you actually have full-blown poisoning.

Checking for toxins is a matter of looking at other body fluids. We use an assortment of tests from several different companies to evaluate your potential toxin levels in your waste because your body is programmed to eliminate toxins there. So we'll do what's called a provoked urine test for heavy metals. Obviously, if you're storing toxins, then that means you're not getting rid of them. So we give you a substance that provokes them to get moving, so they can be bound and excreted. Then you pee and send your urine in for analysis.

We'll also do a urine test for mycotoxins, pesticides, and environmental toxins. Many times, we'll use glutathione or another nutrient to mobilize the mold toxins in the body so you can see it when it comes out. We may also encourage you to use a sauna or Epsom salt bath to help boost that mobilization.

Remember earlier when I used the spigot analogy to talk about getting toxins out? You actually have to ramp up your body's ability to detox and get the toxins moving before you can really see what's actually present. The process can feel discouraging. People often ask us, "Why didn't I see it on my first test?" The answer is often because their ability to detox, like mine, was impaired. When they retest and can see the toxins, it actually means their body's ability to release them is improving.

When I did my provoked tests for metals, I barely looked positive. But after sixteen months of detoxing, I'm finally seeing them move. Unfortunately, it's just not a linear process. Retesting and reacting to the data obtained is a critical part of the process.

Results

Frankly, if you've reached the stage where you're getting the tests run, then you probably won't be surprised to find you have toxins in you. What may be surprising is to find to what extent and which toxins.

If you have toxins, your doctor will custom tailor a protocol just for you. And, again, plan on retesting. Especially with metals and environmental toxins. When removing the metals ("detoxing"), you will also pull out nutrients you need to be healthy. So you must regularly retest to ensure you are not overtreating. Of course, while doing your metals detox, you will also need to replace the typical nutrients lost with supplementation.

Retesting and supplementation will be just part of your plan to get clean. But you know what? You may discover your whole life will need to be examined and potentially overhauled. So, up next, we're going to talk about how to get clean!

Hot Top Tips

1. Inventory your symptoms (and don't just chalk them up to aging!). (Complete the symptom questionnaire earlier in this chapter to get your toxicity score.)

2. Get a Functional Medicine evaluation.

3. Evaluate your overall health.

4. Clean up your diet.

5. Balance your microbiome.

6. Dive into the toxins evaluation when you're ready!

CHAPTER 8

This Girl Is on Fire!

My patient Megan is an ICU nurse who showed up in my office in December wrapped up in a coat and scarf, wearing a hat and giant sunglasses. Aside from the sunglasses, her attire wasn't abnormal for a Massachusetts winter; however, as she peeled back the layers, I realized she wasn't just protecting herself from the cold. She was hiding as much of her skin as possible so people wouldn't stare at her. Megan was covered from head to toe with a red, scaly, itchy rash. In addition, after interviewing her, I learned about her debilitating exhaustion, inability to sleep, out-of-control anxiety, irritable bowel, and brain fog.

The rash was eczema, and it literally covered her from head to toe. Her hands were scaly and cracked. Her face was red, inflamed, and flaky. And the rash was even in her vagina! The girl was on fire! But not in a good way. Megan hated leaving the house, was struggling in her job—and sex? It was too painful for her to even think about. She felt so crappy and hated how

141

she looked so much that she had broken up with her boyfriend and had quit socializing with friends. But she was hoping there would be a quick fix, since she was leaving for Disney in three weeks with her family.

Now, I'm good, but...miracles take time! So the first thing I told her was that a three-week turnaround to amazing health was neither possible nor realistic, and we were looking at a six-month runway (at the very least!). I told her up front that I suspected toxins because she was the second patient I'd seen with such an intense rash accompanied by the same sleep problems and mental fogginess, so we began there.

It's pretty rare that people are too sick to work, but Megan was. As an ICU nurse, she really needed to be at the top of her game, and not sleeping, brain fog, extreme fatigue, and her embarrassment over her rash were all impairing her performance. So, while we were starting the workup, one of the things I recommended was a leave of absence from work so she could focus exclusively on getting better. Her health really was that bad.

As part of the initial interventions, I had her eliminate all processed foods from her diet and eat only clean, organic foods. And we tested her for metals and molds. Her mercury levels came back as positive. She was negative for lead and had multiple strains of mycotoxins in her. So we began a full-fledged detox program.

Megan was super motivated and really wanted to get back to work (and fix her skin!), so she dove into her treatment regimens and changed her entire diet and lifestyle along with the treatments. Within a few weeks, her sleep quality improved, her anxiety lessened, and her gut function normalized. Fast-forward a few months and her skin started clearing up, her energy increased, and she felt she was thinking clearly enough to go back to work. She wasn't done with her treatment by any stretch of the imagination, but she was steadily improving.

Just a comment about her skin; it's really hard to understate how bad it was. When I say that "her skin was clearing up," I mean that her face was no longer bright red and flaky, her hands were no longer cracked and bloody, and she was developing normal skin in these areas. She wasn't "done," but her skin quality had significantly improved after only a few months. She was still wearing long sleeves and pants but no longer felt the need to cover up every bit of skin, and she was willing to go out without a scarf and sunglasses.

During metals removal, we retested frequently to gauge where she was so we could stop treatment when she was done. For Megan, as it is with many people, her body released metals at different rates. As we continued the treatment, when her mercury levels started going down, we noticed lead appearing. To go back to the rusty spigot analogy, even when it's cranked wide open, not everything can come through it at once. Similarly, one of the things that makes detox a bit tricky is that your body can't show or release everything at the same time. So as there was less mercury in her body to eliminate, there became room in her pathways to start releasing the lead.

The really cool thing is that we have a happy ending to this story. Megan came in last summer, about eighteen months after her first visit.

"Look at you in your tank top and short shorts!" I greeted her. "You've got it all going on! Holy smokes, you look amazing!"

Her skin had completely cleared up; she was perky and feeling vibrant. She was dating again and no longer uncomfortable in her own skin. And did I mention she was back at work and doing amazing? Because that's what being clean is all about.

What's a Girl Gotta Do to Get Clean around Here?

As Megan's story illustrates, detoxing often takes a whole-lifestyle approach. The ultimate goal is to reduce your exposure as you increase your removal. This involves being strategic in your food choices, taking supplements prescribed by your doctor, making lifestyle changes, and possibly altering your environment and your relationships.

Detoxification is a two-phase process, but there are some things that we recommend you do as part of your overall detox experience. We've put together a list of food-related changes that you can make to begin improving your health immediately.

- Completely eliminate:

    * All refined or processed foods and beverages. This includes bread, pasta, pastries, tortillas, cookies, candies, soda, and juices made from concentrate.

    * All processed or packaged grains (both with gluten or gluten-free) including crackers, chips, and other snack foods

    * Foods that list any of the following in the ingredients: cane sugar, honey, maple syrup, coconut sugar, corn syrup, or any other form of sugar (even if it's organic)

    * Gluten in any form, whether from wheat, barley, rye, or oats that are not certified as gluten-free

    * High-GMO foods like those containing processed corn or corn derivatives like maltodextrin, dextrose, or dextrin

    * Dairy foods, especially those that are processed or made from nonorganic cow's milk (including yogurt, cheese, cream, cream cheese, butter, and ice cream)

    * Caffeine and alcohol (though one to two cups of green tea is okay)

- Eat lots of:

    * Veggies! Try to get seven to ten servings of vegeta-
      bles a day (a serving size is one half cup cooked or
      one cup raw).

    * Microgreens or sprouts. Sprouts from arugula,
      broccoli, and sunflowers have ten to twenty times
      the nutrition of their larger counterpart.

    * Healthy plant-rich fats like olive, olive oils, raw
      nuts, seeds, avocados, and coconuts

    * Grass-fed beef, organic, free-range poultry, and
      wild-caught (low-mercury) seafood and shellfish

    * Organic, free-range whole eggs

    * Low-sugar fruits—blueberries, strawberries, rasp-
      berries, and other berries as well as green apples

    * Organic starchy vegetables—sweet potatoes,
      carrots, beets, and starchy squashes like butternut,
      kabocha, delicata, and spaghetti (Yes, white pota-
      toes can be eaten, but only in season and organic,
      otherwise choose the purple ones.)

    * Sea vegetables—seaweed or seasonings made from
      them, such as Maine Coast Sea Vegetables Dulse,
      kelp seasonings, and Eden Foods' Gomasio

- Eat these in moderation:

    * Packaged grain-free foods (e.g., Simple Mills brand of crackers or Siete tortillas)—but keep them to one small portion a day.

    * Gluten-free whole grains such as brown, black, or wild rice and quinoa—but limit the quantity to no more than a half cup per meal.

    * Non-GMO/organic soy may be eaten in its whole-food forms (tofu, edamame, and minimally processed, unsweetened soy milks) three to five times a week.

    * Corn, if you can find it non-GMO and in season

    * Sheep-, goat-, or buffalo-milk-based dairy as a "condiment"—meaning a sprinkling or a dollop of yogurt—if you know you tolerate it well.

    * Plant-based dairy alternatives based on nuts, as long as they do not contain added sugars, canola oils, soybean oils, or inorganic soy additives.

- Related to your food intake, consider:

    * Intermittent fasting, where you only eat within a twelve- to eighteen-hour window every day (only drinking water the remaining time)

    * Stay hydrated! Speaking of water, aim for about
    half your body weight in ounces. Can't stand it
    plain? Squeeze in a little lemon or lime juice or try
    plain seltzer or organic herbal teas. And to make
    your water even more of a hydrator, drop in some
    electrolyte tabs.

Again, remember, all the above points are strategies to support your overall detox program. When your lab results come back saying you do have a toxic body burden, we'll recommend you do more than just the above. See, there are particular foods that actually upregulate bodily detoxification, meaning they will help get the toxins out of you.[44] In addition to those particular foods, there are supplements that will assist as well. Exactly what kind will depend on what's in your body.

You see, heavy metals require a different approach than mold does, and both of them need something different than detoxing for environmental toxins and pesticides. However, we often find that if you have one toxin, you have others; remember, it comes down to a common pathway, which makes you ineffective at detoxing in general, so you get a buildup. Then if you have more than one kind of toxin in your body and you want to address them simultaneously, that can mean you take a *lot* of supplements!

---

44   Romilly E. Hodges and Deanna M. Minich, "Modulation of Metabolic Detoxification Pathways Using Foods and Food-Derived Components: A Scientific Review with Clinical Application," *Journal of Nutrition and Metabolism* (2015), www.ncbi.nlm. nih.gov/pmc/articles/PMC4488002/; J. C. Cline, "Nutritional Aspects of Detoxification in Clinical Practice," Alternative Therapies in Health and Medicine 21, no. 3 *(2015): 54–62,* https://pubmed.ncbi.nlm.nih.gov/26026145/.

Ed and I have designed detox programs around food that work in accordance with how your body naturally detoxes. Our approach will improve your liver's ability to get rid of toxins, help bind and remove the toxins from your body, and replace any minerals or nutrients that may be lost during your detox. And all of that is in alignment with the two phases of detoxification.

Detox: The Two-Step Tango

Detox happens in two phases, and there are particular foods and supplements that help with each one. Trust me, you wouldn't be the first person to look over the list of foods for each phase and think, *Geesh, that's a lot of vegetables and stuff. Can't I just take a few more supplements, like some multivitamins or something, instead of eating all that food?*

And the answer is not really. There is plenty of research that suggests there is a synergistic aspect to eating a variety of healing foods. They are more powerful when ingested whole than when the phytochemical (the nutrient, like lycopene in tomatoes) is extracted and put it into a pill for you to take. So expect to eat the whole foods for the best results within each phase.

Phase 1

In Phase 1, a group of enzymes in your body (the cytochrome P450 family of enzymes to be exact) converts toxins into smaller substances and then makes the toxins water-soluble so they can enter Phase 2. Part of that conversion process requires oxidation to happen, which can mean free radicals are released. That's not a good thing. If free radicals get to run rampant in your body, they can cause disease and even cancer. So this phase is all about getting things prepped and in position to move *out* of the body quickly.

To support this phase, we encourage foods and supplements that provide antioxidants to fight off the free radicals and assist in the binding. It's a multi-pronged approach!

- Supplements (as a starting point; your individual situation will determine exact supplements):

    * Vitamins A, B, C, and E

    * Minerals magnesium, selenium, copper, zinc, manganese, and iron

    * Lipotropics (in particular methionine, choline, cysteine, and inositol), which are compounds that break down fat

- Foods that support Phase 1:

    * Carrots, winter squash, kale, sweet potatoes, raw tomatoes (high in beta carotenes)

    * Citrus juices and peels, strawberries (rich source of vitamin C and bioflavonoids)

    * Spinach (high in B vitamins)

    * Sunflower seeds (good source of vitamin E and calcium)

* Brazil nuts (high in selenium)

* Mussels (one of the best sources of zinc and trace minerals)

* Garlic, chives, leeks, onions (high in thiols)

* Cruciferous vegetables such as broccoli, cauliflower, brussels sprouts, cabbage, turnips, collard greens, kale, bok choy (high in sulforaphane and glutathione, especially when eaten raw)

* Blueberries (especially wild), pomegranates, blackberries, raspberries, cocoa/cacao (rich source of polyphenols)

* Green tea (high in polyphenols)

* Turmeric and curry (rich in anti-inflammatory compounds called curcuminoids)

Phase 2

In this phase, toxins get conjugated (bound) and then taken out of your body through sweat, urine, and stool. Unfortunately, this phase is usually slower, especially in women. So we put more focus on improving how your body "does" Phase 2. Otherwise, the toxins hang around just waiting to create mischief.

For this phase, we recommend focusing on certain supplements and foods.

- Supplements (as a starting point; your individual situation will determine exact supplements):

  * Glutathione

  * Molybdenum

- Foods containing those same supplements:

  * High-protein foods including grass-fed beef, organic and pastured turkey/chicken, lamb, organ meats such as liver (also rich in vitamin B12)

  * Bone broth, collagen, gelatin (source of trace minerals and amino acids)

  * Eggs, scallops, lobster, crab (high in sulfur)

  * Cilantro and parsley (contain natural chelation agents, high in vitamin A and folate)

  * Pumpkin, carrots, winter squash, dandelion greens (rich in alpha and beta carotenes)

  * Grass-fed whey protein (if tolerated; high in the amino acid L-cysteine, which supports glutathione production)

At this point, your toxins are bound and ready to be released in your stool, urine, or sweat. That means adequate hydration is a must, so you can pee and sweat them out. Ginger can also be helpful in this stage, as it stimulates digestion and sweating.

It's vital that you do not get constipated! If toxins (and remember, hormones are toxins!) are just sitting there in your stool that is not moving, they can easily get recycled and be put back into your body.

Something important to remember is that hormones that have been processed and are on their way out of your body can also get recycled. It happens in your gut and is worse if you're constipated or have particularly high levels of the enzyme that unbinds the estrogens. These hormones, though produced in your body, can be quite toxic, particularly estrogen. They need to be excreted!

This is why, many times, we recommend substances that improve how often you have a bowel movement, such as magnesium, fiber, enemas, medium-chain triglyceride (MCT) oil and other substances that make pooping easier and more regular.

Elimination

You could consider elimination the third phase of detoxification. As just mentioned, you eliminate toxins through urine, stool, and sweat. Steam rooms and exercise are great ways to get the poisons out via sweat. So are saunas.

I now sit in a sauna almost every day. In fact, because we didn't take a vacation this year, due to COVID-19, we bought a sauna for our home. In addition to making you sweat, infrared saunas are designed to reach the cellular level, so they actually promote the removal of toxins in the cells.

Saunas don't have to require a home makeover. You can find relatively inexpensive ones on Amazon, Sharper Image, or Wayfair. They can look like a sort of pod that you zip yourself into. What's most important when purchasing one of these—or if you have a sauna built into your home—is that you get one that has low EMFs. You'll need to do some research to find that out. And if you purchase one of the pod types, it will probably be made from vinyl, so you'll want to let it off-gas for a while before you use it.

> Steam helps with detox, too, as well as with congestion, so it can be quite useful. However, it does not penetrate deep into the tissues the way a sauna will.

Saunas are great, but have you ever heard of float tanks or salt tanks? Yeah, I know, some people think they are all woo-woo, but floatation therapy can be very beneficial when it comes to detoxing. Epsom salts are the primary salt they use in the tanks.

They assist in elimination by helping pull toxins out of your body. Epsom salts are also rich with magnesium, so your whole body relaxes, giving you some stress relief too. You don't have to go to a spa to do an Epsom salt bath either; you can do a full-body soak or even a foot bath from the comfort of your home!

One way to improve elimination through sweat is to improve your blood circulation. Body techniques such as dry brushing and cupping are great for that. Dry brushing is the practice of rubbing a brush with stiff bristles against your skin in a circular motion. Cupping will also get circulation moving. Cupping is a form of traditional Chinese medicine. Acupuncturists often do it by applying heat on the backside of a glass pressed against you to create a suction effect that pulls up on your skin. There are now silicone kits you can buy to use at home that will work in a similar way.

We can't end a discussion on elimination without talking about sleep. Yes, sleep. When we sleep, there is a mechanism—we don't know what it is, exactly—that drains toxins and waste products from your brain. Your sleeping brain even gets rid of toxic proteins that are implicated in Alzheimer's. It does this by shrinking your brain cells by about 60 percent so that the space between the cells can be flushed out.

You may have noticed we've mentioned sleep several times in this book. And you probably don't need us to tell you that getting the proper amount of sleep is important—we all know that. But do you know why it's so important?

Aside from detoxing your brain, sleep is when your body repairs and rebuilds your muscles and recuperates. By not sleeping well, or not sleeping enough, you drain and strain your body. The stress of not sleeping increases your cortisol levels.

Interestingly, many of the medications that help people sleep don't allow for the full range of sleep patterns. When you fall asleep under the influence of a prescription medication, you do not go through all the cycles of sleep that your body needs and therefore do not recover as well.

This also goes for alcohol and caffeine. Many people state that they can fall asleep after drinking a cup of coffee, and that is definitely true. However, studies show that the quality of their sleep is significantly reduced.

Now that you see how detox is really a two-phase process (really three if you include the elimination part), let's look at what else your Functional Medicine doctor may suggest you do as part of your detoxification program. First up for that will be making sure your microbiome is healthy and stays healthy.

Fixing the Microbiome

The best way to repair your microbiome and bring it into a healthy balance is by eating a clean diet. That means:

- Choose organic foods and avoid vegetables and fruits that have been grown with pesticides.

- Forget the booze and coffee, and drink water and tea—but never from plastic bottles. Again, one to two cups of green tea is fine, and for some people a small amount of organic coffee (make sure it's mold-free and don't add milk or sugar!) can also be beneficial.

- Eliminate dairy and grains as much as you can, and make sure they're organic when you do eat them!

- We said it earlier in this chapter, but it's so important: you must ditch the processed carbs! We're talking white flour, white rice, and anything that comes in a sealed bag or box. Organic or not, these are not healthy for your gut! Part of the danger of processed foods is that often they are packaged in materials that are toxic—even organic foods! So, if by chance you *do* tolerate wheat very well and you *do* purchase only organic pasta, it's *very* possible your macaroni has ortho-phthalates in it.[45]

---

45   Michael Corkery, "Annie's Pledges to Purge a Class of Chemicals from Its Mac and Cheese," *New York Times*, February 19, 2021, www.nytimes.com/2021/02/19/business/annies-mac-cheese-plastic-phthalates.html.

- Limit sugar intake—especially if anything has more than eight grams of sugar per serving!

- When you eat meats, choose from grass-fed beef (or grass-finished); organic, free-range poultry; and wild-caught fish (and you'll need to avoid tuna, swordfish, mahi-mahi, Chilean sea bass, and the other large predatory fish because they are very high in mercury).

Did you see the movie *Super Size Me*? In it, Morgan Spurlock did a social experiment. He ate nothing but McDonald's for thirty days. The results were drastic changes in his physical, emotional, and psychological health. Drastic changes for the worse. He did quite a bit of damage to his liver, cholesterol, and gut microbiome.

For comparison, studies have been done on thawed-out Neanderthals to look at their microbiome. As you might imagine, they had a pretty clean diet. What was discovered is that our human ancestors had the same strains of intestinal flora as we do today. But in their guts, the ratios of the different bacteria were significantly different.

So which do you think is the best approach? The modern fast-food diet or a clean diet?

In Chapter 9, we'll go into more detail on why the above are the best foods to eat—and we'll discuss the ones to eliminate—in order to get and stay clean. In short: they're what your microbiome needs and wants to thrive. And a thriving gut needs a healthy balance of bacteria, which, for some of us, means we need to add probiotics to our diet too.

You're probably familiar with probiotics: they are the good bacteria in cultured foods like yogurt that help strengthen your immune system. Other sources of this good bacteria are a variety of other fermented foods like kimchi, fermented pickles, and kombucha. But do be careful when buying kombucha and yogurt, and read the labels carefully. Many, even the organic items, are loaded with sugar! Sugar will feed the bad bacteria and yeast, which means there will be little, if any, positive effects from the good bacteria in your gut.

If your microbiome is really out of whack, you may need more than just the right foods to help it get into shape. Some people have such a bad disruption in their gut that they develop a condition called small intestinal bacterial overgrowth (SIBO). People who take antibiotics are at risk for SIBO, along with people who are suffering from significant stress or have a poor diet, low stomach acid, celiac disease, Crohn's, or other major health events. Unfortunately, while we are advanced enough in the medical world to know we need a healthy microbiome with diverse bacteria, we are only now discovering that the microbiome is constantly changing throughout our lives. The diverse ratios you needed five to ten years ago are different than what you need now. Because of that, we recommend changing whatever kind of probiotic you are taking every six months or so, in order to give your gut a good variety.

There is a word of warning concerning *Lactobacillus* and *Bifido-bacterium* probiotics. There are people who cannot tolerate either because their bacterial makeup is so imbalanced. For these folks, those probiotics may worsen their condition. In that case, we encourage spore-based probiotics (the *Bacillus* species). The spore-based probiotics will kill the bad bacteria and make room for the good to grow.

Often when we talk about the microbiome and getting a healthy stomach, many people ask us about gastroesophageal reflux disease, or GERD. What is it, and how does it impact their gut?

What about GERD?

So many people think they have acid reflux problems from having too much stomach acid. And most of them think that because they're on an antacid prescribed by their doctor. However, when we have patients come in complaining of heartburn or indigestion, we don't immediately think they have too much stomach acid. We generally think they don't have enough.

See, when you stack a bunch of toxins and inappropriate bacteria in your microbiome onto aging and an American life filled with stressors, alcohol, anxiety, and sleeplessness, it actually makes your stomach acid levels drop. As you get older, or if you suffer an illness or experience chronic stress, that only worsens the problem of low acidity.

When you have low stomach acid, we say you are experiencing hypochlorhydria. Left to continue, hypochlorhydria can cause constipation, gas, bloating, diarrhea, and malabsorption of vitamins and minerals including folate, B12, calcium, iron, and magnesium. It can also contribute to iron-deficiency anemia, dry and thin skin and hair, acne, dysbiosis (the improper balance of gut bacteria), allergies, chronic fatigue, bone loss/ osteoporosis, and a weakened immune system. However, the most obvious and common symptoms of hypochlorhydria are the exact same as GERD or heartburn.

As you can see, it's important to get the right diagnosis here, because if you treat indigestion due to low stomach acid (hypochlorhydria) with something that suppresses your stomach acid even more, you will worsen the problem *and* your symptoms!

The good news is, it's relatively easy to tell the difference between low stomach acid and high. And you probably have what you need to use to do that in your kitchen: baking soda.

A baking soda solution reacts with your stomach acid to produce carbon dioxide gas. The amount of gas produced depends upon the quantity of acid contained in your stomach. Carbon dioxide makes you burp. When you do this simple test, you will time how long it takes between drinking the baking soda mixture and your burp. The longer it takes, the lower the stomach acid you have. (Be aware: if you are on a PPI [proton pump inhibitor] or any medication that suppresses stomach acid, this test is not going to give you an accurate assessment.)

Here's How to Do
the Stomach Acid Test

- First thing in the morning on an empty stomach (before eating or drinking), dissolve one-quarter teaspoon of baking soda into an eight-ounce glass of cold water.

- Drink all of the solution and start timing.

- Record how long it takes until you first burp.

- Repeat this process for five consecutive days (or longer) at the same time each day to get a solid average for the length of time to burp.

- Compare your results with the following:

  * One minute or less before burp indicates normal acid levels.

  * Between one and two minutes suggests lower-than-normal acid levels.

  * More than two minutes suggests probable hypo-chlorhydria.

Regardless of whether you have GERD, low-stomach acid, or neither, if you want to feel amazing, adequate stomach acid is part of a well-balanced and healthy microbiome, which is imperative for both Phase 1 and Phase 2 of detoxing.

It's funny, using the phrase "Phase 1" or "Phase 2" almost suggests that it's a simple process to detox. Just do this, do that, and heal your gut, then voilà! No more toxins.

Unfortunately, it's not as simple as that. Supplementation alone is quite complex and, honestly, can be quite frustrating. On top of that, remember at the beginning of this chapter when we said detox can require a whole lifestyle makeover? Well, we've only discussed detoxification from the vantage point of looking at what we do on the inside of your body. Let's take a look at what needs to happen outside of your body to get the full benefit of a good detox.

Out-of-Body Experiences

Detox and achieving optimum health requires getting the bad stuff (toxins) out of your body and making sure you have enough of the good stuff (nutrients and hormones) in it. So when you think about it, if you're going through all the trouble to detox, you don't want to risk adding more toxins at the same time.

So here are a few things you can do in your environment that will help your detox efforts.

Air

After you have an appointment with us, we might recommend getting an air quality test on your home. Home Depot sells kits to test for mold for around ten dollars. However, if your budget allows, we'd recommend doing some research in your local area to find a qualified company to come in and do a full evaluation of your home.

To test your air, look for a kit or a company that will test for:

- Mold

- Allergens like dust, dander, pollen, and dust mites

- Volatile organic compounds (VOCs), which include formaldehyde, lead, and radon

- Other pollutants that they might recommend

Now, if you live near a major highway, airport, or a farm that's frequently sprayed with pesticides, herbicides, and fungicides, you shouldn't be surprised by unwelcome air quality results. You may want to consider moving. But if you can't afford to, or if you don't live in one of those places and have high results of toxins on the results anyway, you'll want to invest in a HEPA air filter system. And, of course, then implement filters or other treatments to help alleviate any issues discovered on the test. Most companies will provide you with a list of recommendations based on their results. Don't be afraid to ask!

Something to keep in mind about air (and water) quality test-ing is that yes, those tests can be helpful: however, you do have to take them with a grain of salt because a negative result only means *right now* there are no toxins. A negative result on the home you live in *now* doesn't reflect your childhood home, the dank basement apartment you had in grad school, or even your car. Yes, I had a patient whose car was in a flood and had become moldy. She had to sell her car in order to completely detox from the mold.

Speaking of cars, if you happen to live outside of New Jersey, where it's actually against the law to pump your own gas, it's worth paying the slightly higher price for full service at gas stations. Do not expose yourself to the gas fumes and risk them lingering on your clothing.

Water

If you're toxic, we may suggest getting a water test run as well as an air one. If you have water supplied by your municipality, they should have information on their website telling you what their testing shows. However, if you get one run on your home faucet, you may find more toxins.

The *New York Times* recently did a review of several home water testing kits.[46] According to them, the best one out there is the Simple Water Tap Score test (www.mytapscore.com).

---

46 Tim Heffernan, "The Best Water Quality Test Kit for Your Home," New York Times, February 7, 2020, www.nytimes.com/wirecutter/reviews/best-water-quali-ty-test-kit-for-your-home/.

To use the test, you simply fill some vials of water from your sink and send them off. The testing company examines it and provides a report that looks for more than a hundred different compounds, including:

- Lead

- Mercury

- Arsenic

- VOCs, including chloroform

- Bacteria

- Pesticides

- Nitrites

While MyTap does offer chlorine tests with each of their kits, do consider purchasing their add-on test for perchlorate.

Keep Good Company

Once you know what's going on in the air around you or possibly lurking in the water you're drinking and bathing in, it will be time to give yourself a long look inward. Ask the hard questions about your relationships with yourself and others.

Do you have confidence? Do you trust yourself to make good decisions? How do you talk about and to yourself? Do you ever say things like "God! I'm such an idiot!"? Even in jest, negative self-talk can make your cortisol levels go up.

Being surrounded by negative, toxic people will too. We said it earlier, but I want to reinforce it here: you cannot detox your physical body and maintain toxic relationships. Soul-sapping people who don't uplift you, who don't support you, and who don't believe in you are bad for your health! You do not deserve to be treated that way!

As part of your detox protocol, you may need to learn to set boundaries—or hire a professional to teach you. Probably five times a year, I find myself telling a patient, "I'm sorry. I cannot help you. We have some really cool tools to fix your body, but they will be useless as long as you stay in _____" (whatever the relationship is: a marriage, job, "friendship," or something else).

Yes, cleaning up your life can be a lot of work! I know. I'm living it, which means I know you can do it too! It is possible.

Detox in Real Life

Let's see what this all looks like in real life. In my case, I would roll out of bed and take my mold binders (two pills each of four different ones—yep, eight pills first thing in the morning). Then I'd putter around, get my kids up, exercise, shower, and take some more supplements along with a portion of the metals protocol. On my way into work, I would take a metals treatment. Around eleven o'clock in the morning, I'd often eat breakfast and take all my regular supplements. Lunch would happen around one o'clock, and I'd take more detox supplements. Sometime around three o'clock in the afternoon, I'd take another mold dose, because I wasn't eating anything at that time and those need to be taken on an empty stomach. Before I left the office, I'd take a dose of the metals protocol.

As soon as I would get home from work, I'd take more of the metals protocol treatments and more supplements with dinner. At bedtime, to ramp up elimination, I'd sit in a sauna and take more supplements that bind to toxins. I'd also do a steam every day (and sometimes twice!).

Now, keep in mind, because I have such terrible absorption, I need to take a lot of supplements in general. So, from the general health and detox needs, at one point I was taking anywhere from thirty-five to forty pills a day! At the end of ten months, I was about to explode. I just couldn't take it anymore. So I stopped my mold treatment. Bad patient! I know!

When I retested, I saw that one of the mold toxins, the ochratoxin, had gone up from 20 on the first testing to 146! Yep, the testing showed even more mold in me! It's not as discouraging as it sounds, though. It meant all the binders I was taking, my regular sweaty exercise, and the steaming were working. My body was pulling the toxins out of the storage depots and making it available to be eliminated. And, despite the ochratoxin and another strain increasing, I saw that I had eliminated two other strains completely.

Same thing happened for the metals protocol. Remember how I started out with pretty low levels? Well, each time I've retested after completing a round, the lead and mercury levels came back *higher*! Discouraging in one sense, since I'd like it to be *done*, but encouraging from the standpoint of seeing that the toxins are finally moving.

On a positive, note, I just retested my environmental toxins and glyphosate levels after six months; the glyphosate is now undetectable, and *five* of the environmental toxins that were near or above the seventy-fifth percentile are now significantly lower! Just like with metals and molds, if you test before they're gone, the numbers will look higher, and that's the case for three additional toxins in my environmental toxins report, so I'm continuing to focus on sauna and detox. I really needed that good news, since I've felt frustrated at how difficult it's been to get rid of my metals.

So anyway...I went back on the protocols for toxins, mold, and metals. I may have lost count at this point, but I'm on my fifth or sixth round of the metals detox. Because I'm one of the people who apparently holds onto their toxins(!), we've made the metals protocol successively more intense each time I come back higher.

The thing is, it's tiring to detox! So I sleep more, but that doesn't mean that I sleep five hours a night when I'm not detoxing. I still sleep seven to eight when I'm not detoxing. I sleep eight or more when I'm detoxing because I need the rest.

And so far we've only discussed supplements and sweat! I also eat a very clean diet, and I have my home and work environments set up to be as nontoxic as possible.

Detox is a lot of work! But it's *so* worth it!

Over the last year or so, as I've worked on my own detox, I've been so happy to see some pretty noticeable changes. For one thing, I feel sharper mentally. I mean, we have four kids and two businesses. Ours is a busy household, and we have lots of local family, so I often feel pulled in a million different directions. Frequently, before the detox efforts, I found I couldn't keep track of the details of everything going on around me. A year or so ago, way too many people were saying things to me like "I told you this already" or "I can't believe you forgot that!" Now that's not happening as much.

Other exciting news is that I've lost weight! I'd been working out five to seven days a week for about three years. For the first year, all I did was get fatter—and don't tell me *muscle weighs more than fat*. I was fatter, not more muscle-y. However, the fat has shrunk and *now* I'm building some muscle. I look better in my clothes. And the uncontrollable food cravings and appetite I've had over the past couple of years are just gone.

But best of all? My hair is growing back! I look like a mess because of all the new hair growth, but I keep reminding myself that "mess" is good news!

So yeah! I look good and feel freaking fantastic! But you know what? I don't think I would have made it this far without the support and help from Ed and the entire staff at Five Journeys. Detoxing is not the easiest thing to do. So please don't go it alone.

No woman is an island. We all need support.

Whether it's a group of girlfriends all interested in taking this journey with you, the loving support of your partner and family, or a Functional Medicine practitioner like Ed or me—or all of the above—lean on them. Rely on their help. Put away the Superwoman (or Superman) cape and let them help you. And really, if you think about it, the whole world helped you become toxic. So why wouldn't you rely on a little help to detox?

Hot Top Tips

1. Improve your foods: *in*crease organic foods and veggies and *de*crease your processed foods and sugars.

2. Support Phase 1 and 2 detox:

   a. See the detox list of foods.

   b. Decrease alcohol.

3. Poop. Every day. Or more!

4. Love your gut:

   a. Balance the microbiome.

   b. Increase your probiotics.

   c. Test your stomach acid.

5. Test your air and water in your home.

6. Be kind to yourself.

7. Get the support of the people in your life. With whom do you have the best relationship? Call that person, thank them for always having your back, and tell them about your plans to detox.

CHAPTER 9

A Clean Girl in a Dirty World!

As you can see below, I still have a little way to go before I can say I'm completely toxin-free, but I'm getting cleaner every day. I continue to remove my toxins and reduce my total body amount of them.

But as I described at the end of the last chapter, I'm already seeing positive results from all the detoxing I'm currently doing. I mean...my hair is growing back! Obviously, removing toxins is important, but...growing back my hair is life changing. 🫠

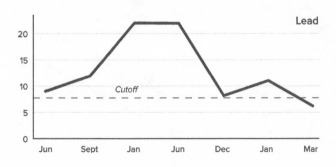

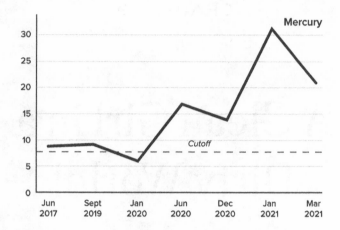

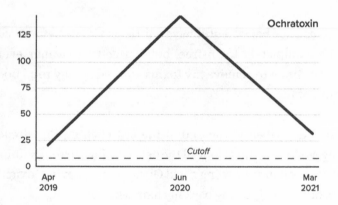

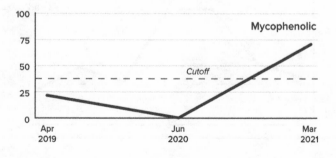

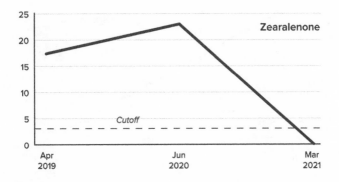

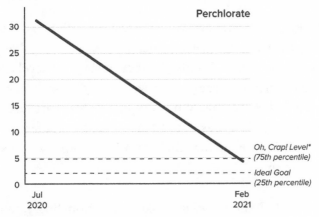

*We recommend treatment when data points are higher than the 75th percentile.

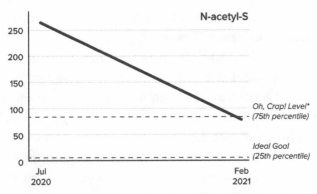

*We recommend treatment when data points are higher than the 75th percentile.

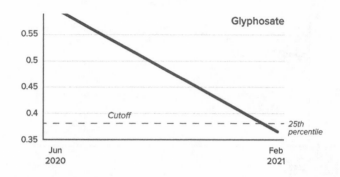

So now my job, as with everyone else who gets clean, is to keep my body as clean as possible, which isn't exactly easy. We live in a very dirty world! Avoiding and removing low-level exposures is a constant struggle that we all must fight inside our homes as well as outside. While I've known for years just how toxic our world is, it wasn't until just this past summer that I experienced firsthand how difficult it is to keep my exposure to a minimum.

Due to COVID-19, we didn't take a vacation this summer. So, since the whole family was spending most of their time at home, we decided to finish our basement. When we discussed our needs and wants with our contractor, we insisted that he use nontoxic materials. Now, many people will say they build "green" or use "eco-friendly" materials. And that's great. But just because something is good for the environment doesn't mean that it is nontoxic! You may need to insist on reading the material safety data sheets (MSDSs) to be sure you're building or renovating with products that are nontoxic. Manufacturers are required to provide an MSDS for every product they make that may be of environmental or health concern. If you cannot find the MSDS easily on the web, then give the company a call.

It was easy to get our contractor to use non-VOC paints and stains. VOC stands for volatile organic compounds. Aside from common sense telling you to stay away from anything labeled *volatile*, let *me* tell you to stay away from paints with VOCs. Those are the ones that produce a lot of chemicals in the air. That fresh paint smell? Think of it like an overabundance of aftershave or perfume on an otherwise attractive person flirting with you—it's a sure sign to stay away!

VOCs are chemicals that can cause short- and long-term health problems.[47] They are often found in paints, varnishes, refrigerants, and even pharmaceuticals. Because VOCs are such a problem, it is relatively easy to find paints without them, but they may cost a little more.

However, as the saying goes, the devil is in the details, and we got tripped up by a few of them! Our plumber apparently didn't get the message that he needed to use nontoxic materials. Subsequently, the glues he used on the pipes were flat-out awful! I could smell them before I even walked into the house. The glues were so toxic that we had to leave the house for a few hours. Thankfully the smell dissipated pretty quickly, but I was beyond steamed!

As our contractor completed our basement, he did whatever he could to create a nontoxic area. Some products were hard to find, others cost a little more than their toxic counterparts, and even others were in both camps. But still, when we were left

---

47 "What Are Volatile Organic Compounds (VOCs)?" United States Environmental Protection Agency, https://www.epa.gov/indoor-air-quality-iaq/what-are-volatile-organic-compounds-vocs.

with a beautiful basement, we had to leave the windows open for a long while so the area could off-gas. And that's using the cleanest materials we could find!

But we weren't done! Next up was finding furnishings.

Knowing that all of the furniture we could bring in would be treated with flame retardants had me concerned. You can't really leave a sofa out in the elements long enough to off-gas—you'd risk mold making a home on the inside of it!

This is where you'll need to do some sleuthing, and keep in mind that are changing fast. From the time I started looking for furniture to the time we started editing this book (three months-ish), Wayfair added a section on their search to include "sustainability," which means you can sort by the chemicals added to your furniture. That's been super helpful, because you can now decide how clean you want your furniture to be! At the time of editing, Overstock didn't yet offer this feature, but one can hope! However, do know that sometimes furniture is made with organic, green materials and then has a fire-retardant applied to it.

Before this feature launched, I was able to get this information by calling Wayfair; the team there is super helpful, and they sent me options to sort through. It does tend to add a little onto the price, but not as much as you might expect! There are also a number of companies that specialize in organic, chemical-free furniture, although the budget on that is often much larger.

One thing I messed up on was the beanbag chairs I found for my children to use down there. I had a long conversation with the rep and ordered two, feeling pretty confident they would be safe; however, when we opened up the packaging and ripped off the plastic outer coverings, I did notice a chemical smell. There was no way I felt comfortable letting that stuff off-gas down there in a closed space. So, since we weren't having dinner parties either, due to COVID, we put the beanbags in the dining room and opened the windows. That's also the beauty of construction: it always takes longer than anticipated. So...the beanbags went unused for about two months before we were ready to put them in the basement.

So I realize the struggle is real and may never leave. There will always be potential exposures to toxins. Given that, my goal is to remove as many toxins as possible and get my body as healthy as it can be, so that it will not be quite so reactive to whatever exposure I may receive. I also want to make sure I ongoingly support my body's ability to do a better job detoxing in general. And knowing my genes, that may mean I periodically just have to go through another round of detoxing. I know for sure that once I've gotten rid of all of these toxins, I'm not only going to be testing regularly to make sure they're not reaccumulating but also ensuring I support ongoing detox!

However, my situation is not indicative of what it will be like for most people. And after you go through your detox program, you'll be in a better place to figure out what *you* need to do to keep your body clean. Because whether you finish a basement or not, one thing is for sure: you cannot go back to your old dirty habits! If you try to preserve your old lifestyle, you're just going to become toxic again. So plan on making some permanent changes to develop clean habits.

But before you dive in to make changes, ask yourself this question: how do you rip your Band-Aids off?

It's All about Personal Style

You're on the verge of doing a complete overhaul of your life to limit your exposure to possible toxins. It will be a lot to take in and get a handle on, which means it will be easy to give up and go back to your old ways. So why not make it easy on yourself and strategize for how to make these changes come easier to you?

When making any behavioral changes, there are a set of questions to ask first that will help set you up for success:

- Are you a fell-swoop, grand-gesture kind of person? Do you rip your Band-Aids off with one fast flourish? Or are you more prone to incremental steps?

- Are you a self-motivator? That is, once you figure out what you need to do, do you just do it? Or do you need to get support first, some kind of external accountability? If the latter, then you know you'll do better with a coach or a therapist, or someone who will be your accountability buddy.

Getting these basics figured out only gets you halfway there! You have to honor your own style when making changes. The other part that's critical is to ensure that the changes you're making actually *fit* into your life. If you have to eat as soon as you wake up, then you wouldn't want to take a mold treatment right upon waking...you'd want to wait until later! Or if you get a treatment you can't stand the taste or smell of, you'll need to communicate that to your provider so they can make a change! There are *always* substitutions! So remember, if you ever notice yourself struggling or feeling like you're not rocking the treatment, all that means is that you either didn't honor your needs or some components don't match. No worries! Just revisit the questions, tweak your approach, and get back at it!

Now, to get started on cleaning up your lifestyle, why not start with what might be "easy"? And for many that's the food and drinks we consume.

Clean at the Dining Table

Clean Drinking

After reading the previous chapter, you may have had your water tested, or you may still be considering doing it. That test will help you determine whether or not you should have a purifying system installed. My bet is you should. Just about everybody should.

We recommend that you at least get a system to purify your drinking water at the kitchen tap. At the bare minimum, an under-the-counter filtration with a two-part filter will get most of the worst contaminants out of your water. That includes things like mercury, lead, pharmaceuticals, and organic compounds. But a standard filter is not as good as a reverse osmosis system that will eliminate perchlorate and fluoride as well as those others.

While a system that just cleans the water coming through your kitchen sink is good for drinking and cooking, you know that's not your only exposure to water. What's pouring through your shower? What are your little children splashing in when they're in the tub? Do your kids like to splash in a sprinkler on your lawn in the summer? Or—possibly worse—drink from a hose?

For the ultimate in clean water, you can get a system that will service your whole house. Not only that, but you can even find one that, in addition to the filter, has an ultraviolet light to kill bacteria and viruses.

But maybe before you invest in the purification system, you should have a plumber check to see if your plumbing materials are free of lead. Really, that might be a primary concern.

You may think that because your home or fixtures are relatively new, lead in the piping or hardware would be a nonissue. But nope. While there are federal regulations, and states have their own laws on top of those, no one says you *must* make plumbing supplies lead-free.[48] Reread that sentence: no one says you *must* make plumbing supplies lead-free.

---

48 At the time of this writing, President Biden's American Jobs Plan includes $45 billion to eliminate lead pipes and service lines in the United States. "Fact Sheet: The American Jobs Plan," White House, March 31, 2021, https://www.whitehouse. gov/briefing-room/statements-releases/2021/03/31/fact-sheet-the-american-jobs-plan/.

And of the companies that do make "lead-free" products, most often abide by the legal definition of that phrase, which says *a faucet can leach lead into water* up to eleven parts per billion.[49]

Sure, that's probably safe for a one-time exposure. Or a couple exposures over an extended period of time. Possibly even for everyday exposure for someone who has a healthy microbiome and good MTHFR genes. But what about the rest of us? What about those of us struggling with a body on the brink of too many toxins? Really, is any exposure to lead safe? I don't think so.

Now, what can you do about your pipes and supplies? One way to know if yours are "safe" according to federal regulations is to find the packaging they came in and see if there is a stamp on it that says "NSF 61/9." Don't have the packaging? Who does, right? You might then have to do some research with the manufacturer to get the information. If there is no NSF 61/9 stamp, but you do find a Proposition 65 warning for the state of California, then the product may have lead or other toxins in it. (The folks who live in California are a little luckier than the rest of us, in that they have some of the strictest laws in the country regarding toxins.) So try to find a replacement.

Keep in mind that the above information is only for faucets that supply drinking water. That coding is not required or mandated to be on hose bibs, bathtub fixtures, shower heads, or industrial faucets. Federal and state lead regulations do not apply to them. Go figure.

49 "Lead in Drinking Water," Centers for Disease Control and Prevention, November 18, 2020, https://www.cdc.gov/nceh/lead/prevention/sources/water.htm.

Say No to Plastic!

While we're on the subject of water, it's time to quit drinking from single-use bottles: water, sodas, fruit juices, kombucha, or any other drink that comes in a single-use bottle. Even if the label claims there is no BPA in the packaging, the plastics still leach into the water and then you drink them. *All plastic comes from petroleum products.* They are endocrine disruptors, which you might remember means they will f*ck—I mean, they will mess up your hormones!

So don't buy water, juice, milk, or anything else that is housed in a plastic container. Don't store your foods in plastic either. And for heaven's sake, don't heat up or microwave anything that is in a plastic container! The hotter the food or drink, the more plastic will melt into it.

Yes, that means throw out the Keurig! Think about it: it heats water up and then forces it through a plastic container into your cup.

Now that you're potentially shocked and disturbed to find that two of your most frequently used items are a no-go (single-use plastic and Keurig coffee), maybe I should forewarn you: you're about to get potentially more bad news: it's time to divorce sugar.

Cut Out Sugar

Sugar is like a sexy hoodlum in a black leather jacket leaning against a motorcycle. You make eye contact. You receive a slight nod in acknowledgment. You go weak in the knees and float over just to say hello. Your girlfriends are simultaneously jealous and worried as they see you indulge, and...well, ahem. So, yes, sugar is sweet and delightful. But it's also like that leather-clad biker...loaded with trouble!

The thing about sugar is that, really, it's both a matter of quantity *and* quality. If you come to us and say you have a teaspoon of organic honey in your hot tea every day, we're not going to go crazy. However, most people are not conscious of how much sugar they are actually eating. I once had a patient who came to me with a body that was completely out of whack. She couldn't believe her diet had anything to do with it because it was so clean. She ate loads of fresh fruit and vegetables every day—including two five-pound bags of mandarin oranges a day! Yes, two bags!

Four mandarin oranges would be two servings of fruit for one day. She was far exceeding that number and overloading her poor body with fructose sugar.

Sugar is sugar, even if it comes from a Cutie or a Meanie mandarin orange. Thankfully, once she cut back, her body rebounded beautifully.

So be aware of how much sugar is in everything. The recommended dietary allowance (RDA) for sugar is forty grams a day. Do you know how many grams of sugar are in one can of Coke? Thirty-nine! (Not to mention all the other ugly ingredients in it.)

Not-so-fun fact: the sugar that makes up those thirty-nine grams in a twelve-ounce can of Coke comes from high-fructose corn syrup (HFCS). Do you know what the least innocent sugar is? HFCS. It's not your average bad boy or girl who just wants to take you for a ride on a Harley; it's the one that gets you hooked on drugs. HFCS is linked with so many unhealthy consequences, we could write an entire book about it. Until we do, though, just remember this: HFCS is made from nonorganic corn, which is treated with a sh*t ton of pesticides and herbicides. Then, when the corn is made into syrup, all those toxins become concentrated in the syrup. And don't forget what you read back in Chapter 3—corn syrup has mercury in it! Between the sugar content and the chemicals, you're getting a raw deal.

Look, Ed and I are not inhuman. We totally get it that sometimes sugar can be a special treat. We also get that you live in the real world, and the real world eats sugar! So when we have patients tell us they just cannot eliminate something like chocolate from their lives, we help them rethink their approach to it. Instead of eating an entire candy bar, we suggest you take one square of high-quality dark chocolate and find a quiet place where you'll be undisturbed to eat it. Hide in the broom closet if you have to; you know you are the only one who would ever think to look in there for any reason. Then place the chocolate on the roof of your mouth, close your eyes, and truly savor it.

In short: keep to just thirty-nine grams of sugar a day. It's okay to have a dalliance with the occasional indulgence. Just don't marry the hoodlum. You want someone or something that will treat you right and not cause any hardship. Sugar can't give that to you. But, honestly, it's time to get real. Before you can limit your sugar intake to fewer than forty grams a day, you actually have to know how many grams you're taking in. Prepare to be shocked! But knowing where you stand is the first step to winning this game.

There really is a thing called a sugar addiction. It can be a hard and long process to lose the cravings for sugar. And unfortunately, as with any addiction, if you break the habit and then pick it up again as a "one-time" treat, you'll find it's hard to do just a little bit of sugar. Your body will pick up on it as if you never quit and demand more.

As one of my patients once said, "One is too many and a thousand will never be enough." She's learned for herself that it's not just a slippery slope; it's a greased slide, so she Just. Doesn't. Indulge.

And if all that isn't enough, sugar literally causes you stress! It produces the same physiological effects as emotional stress: indulging in sugar on a regular basis will constantly put your body in a fight-flight-or-freeze mode, which just seems unfair! Who doesn't crave ice cream when they're stressed? It's yet another way stress makes us fat.

Also, remember when we were discussing the microbiome? When your gut is out of balance and you have a yeast over-growth, you will crave sugar, because that's what the yeast needs to survive. The sugar feeds the yeast, which damages your microbiome, which stresses your system, which makes you crave more sugar.

So there are two feedback loops: sugar, stress, anxiety, sugar, stress, anxiety, sugar, stress, anxiety...and sugar, yeast growth, sugar, yeast growth, sugar, yeast growth. Eventually, your body weakens and any predisposition you have for a disease will open a portal for you to develop it.

Yet when you detox from sugar and the brain fog lifts, you'll feel so good you'll be able to resist the temptation to indulge. Just a note here...it takes about two weeks to really get through the sugar addiction, and those two weeks are the hardest! I suggest getting the sugar out of the house during that time frame. Once you've decided to do it, you want to increase the chance of success! If you can't get it out of your house, at least get it out of your line of sight! It's called the "power of suggestion" for a reason!

Steer Clear of Dairy

While we're on the subject of things we love that don't love us back, let's talk about dairy. Look, we're not baby cows. Nor are we baby sheep or goats. Which explains why milk and milk products from those animals are seldom tolerated by humans very well. Dairy is so hard for many of us to digest that it can cause or worsen asthma. It creates phlegm in the body. And it makes skin issues like eczema flare up. Yet here's the crazy thing: it does all that to people who are *not* lactose intolerant! For those poor people who are, the stomach distress dairy causes is just horrible.

Aside from it not being a good option for the human body, the dairy products you find in your market (even the organic ones) have been homogenized to make them safe enough for us to drink. Homogenization is where they take the fat molecules and make them super tiny. Then they pasteurize the milk, which means they heat it up to kill off bacteria. While those processes make a more appetizing and safer product, they also destroy and purge any truly healthy elements of the dairy products. Many of us are really better off just avoiding dairy entirely.

Go Organic

Perhaps it only makes sense at this point that if you are going to have a clean body, you want to have a clean diet. That means go organic as much as possible to eliminate the potential extra toxins from pesticides, herbicides, and fungicides. Unless a food is organic, it can be sprayed with pesticides and herbicides. Fungicides are often sprayed on foods imported into this country, too, so while they may have been grown organically, look on any packaging to see if they have been sprayed with a fungicide.

Aside from the toxins in nonorganic fruits and vegetables, another reason to eat organic ones is that they have better nutrition. Ever hear of phytonutrients? They are the nutrients that are specific to a particular food. Lycopene in tomatoes is a phytonutrient. There are studies that show while the major nutrients (your primary vitamins and minerals) are about the same between nonorganic and organic produce, the phytonutrients differ widely. It's believed that difference is because phytonutrients help a plant defend itself from pests and diseases; plants don't have a chance to develop those muscles when they are sprayed with chemicals.

Phytonutrients are so powerful, they actually tell our genes and our microbiome to turn on anti-inflammatory pathways, and they encourage heart health and immune protection. What's even cooler is that those superpowers are color coded in the foods.[50]

- Red fruits and vegetables contain lycopene, which, among other benefits, is a powerful antioxidant that is believed to protect against certain cancers.

- Orange foods often have beta-carotene, a nutrient your body converts into the vitamin A that it needs.

- Yellow foods contain lutein and zeaxanthin, which are important for eye health.

---

50 Deanna M. Minich, "A Review of the Science of Colorful, Plant-Based Food and Practical Strategies for 'Eating the Rainbow,'" *Journal of Nutrition and Metabolism* (2019), https://doi.org/10.1155/2019/2125070.

- Green foods have a lot of folate in them, otherwise known as vitamin B9. That nutrient is super important for numerous processes in your body: it's required for the production of red and white blood cells, it converts carbohydrates into energy, and it plays an integral role in the production of DNA.

- Blue and purple foods have flavonoids that help regulate cellular activity and are also antioxidants.

The above list is not a completely exhaustive one detailing which nutrients come from which color of food; it's just a beginning. But it clearly demonstrates why it's vital to "eat the rainbow" in terms of natural food colors so you can get the full range of phytonutrients.

To take it a step further, not only should your fruits and vegetables be organic, the meats you eat need to be organic too. Those animals reap the same benefits from organic food as you do, which will make them even healthier for you.

Our recommendations for meat eaters are to choose grass-fed beef first. If it's not available, then look for grass-finished as your next preference, and organic as the third. Regarding poultry, look for free-range, organic poultry. Find pork from humanely raised pigs (stress impacts the quality of their meat). And try to find wild-caught small fish from sustainable sources. By "small" fish, we mean no tuna, swordfish, mahi-mahi, or Chilean sea bass. Those guys usually taste so good because they are fatty, and as the chefs say, "fat is flavor!" But remember, toxins are stored in body fat. That rule applies to fish too. Those species are the ones commonly loaded with mercury and other toxins.

Before we end our discussion on how to have a clean diet, there is one more thing that Ed and I sometimes get pushback on from our clients. And that's alcohol.

Limit the Booze

I know this is one people don't want to hear, but in our opinion, really no amount of alcohol is good for you. Alcohol is, itself, a toxin. And when you drink it, the first thing your liver does is quit paying attention to everything else it's doing to deal with the margarita you're sipping for happy hour. Which means that if there is some toxic sh*t in your body, the alcohol makes your liver too distracted to help you eliminate it.

So, really, whether you truly need to eliminate all alcohol depends on how toxic you are overall. If you're experiencing fatigue, poor sleep, anxiety, hair loss, gut dysfunction, skin issues, or difficulty losing weight, then, yes, cutting it out totally would probably help. But if you're not that sick, you may just want to figure out how much you drink and then cut down by 50 percent.

The type of alcohol matters too. Beer and wine? They are loaded with yeast and convert right to sugar! Vodka? It still stresses the liver and adrenals, but it doesn't jack up the yeast. Sometimes it's about a full reset, and sometimes it's about making an improvement. Again, you know yourself best, so make the choice that is going to work for you in your life!

Question Your Relationship with Gluten and Grains

We've spoken about the negatives related to gluten so much in this book, perhaps it's no surprise that if you want to stay clean, you might be better off keeping gluten out of your diet. Gluten is found in wheat and all of wheat's varieties, including durum, semolina, spelt, farina, farro, graham, einkorn, and so on. Gluten is also found in other grains like rye, barley, triticale, kamut, and malt. It's also in many brewer's yeasts (unless labeled gluten-free) and most wheat starches. Aside from the whole sensitivity thing and opening up your tight junctions, part of the problem with glutinous grains—all grains, really— is that if they are not organic, they probably have glyphosate in them, a weed killer that happens to mess up the microbiome and is a neurotoxin.

Grains often have mold in them, and arsenic has been found in rice! It's just really tough to be a gluten or grain eater *and* have a clean body.

Whew! That was a lot of information to take in, in a short amount of time. But it doesn't have to be an overwhelming process. Take baby steps and move through making dietary changes in phases. Here's a helpful table to guide you through the process:

	ELIMINATE	LIMIT	ADD
LEVEL 1	Artificial colors		
	Artificial flavors		
	Artificial sweeteners		
	Preservatives		
	High-fructose corn syrup		
LEVEL 2	Everything from level 1	Alcohol (one to two drinks per day, max)	Vegetables (aim for three a day)
	Juices (unless self-juiced, then limit amounts)	Caffeine (cut off by 2:00 p.m.; limit to three servings per day)	Healthy fats (olive oil, avocado oil, and coconut oil)
		Snacks— only one or two per day	
		Added sugar	
LEVEL 3	Everything from levels 1 and 2	Fruit—two servings, low-sugar fruits	Vegetables—aim for five servings of organic a day
	Gluten if sensitive; limit if not	Processed carbs	Grass-fed/grass-finished meats
	Dairy if sensitive; limit if not	Added sugars	Ensure healthy fats with meals

	Heavy-mercury fish (check out the EPA guidelines[51])	Unprocessed grains (rice, quinoa, millet, barley, etc.)	
	Alcohol (or significantly limit it)		

Cleaning up your diet will go a long way toward maintaining a clean body. If you need to take a break here as you wrap your thinking around how to incorporate making changes in your diet, do so. And when you're ready, come back and begin Chapter 10. There you'll look at what you can do in your environment to help keep your exposure to toxins at a minimum. Start with one and then move through your diet as you're ready to take on another.

Hot Top Tips

1. Clean up your construction and avoid chemicals!

2. Divorce the single-use plastic bottles.

3. Buy organic!

---

51 "Fish and Shellfish Advisories and Safe Eating Guidelines," United States Environmental Protection Agency, https://www.epa.gov/choose-fish-and-shellfish-wisely/fish-and-shellfish-advisories-and-safe-eating-guidelines.

4. Ditch the sugar.

5. Cut your booze intake by 50 percent.

6. Eliminate processed carbs and gluten.

CHAPTER 10

It's Not Just about Food

L ook, I know it's a big task to live a clean life. And I know this task never ends.

As I make time twice a week to sit with an IV drip as part of my protocol to remove the heavy metals and add antioxidants back into my body, I think about the potentially toxic people and objects in my environment. And every day, I realize there's still something else I need to take care of.

So there's something good that unexpectedly came from my detox! I'm going to continue the habit of reflection on a daily basis. Honestly, I think it's a good idea for everyone to take an inventory of where they spend most of their time to see where they could be getting exposure to invisible toxins in their environment.

To help *you* figure out what kinds of toxins you may be exposed to, we have provided the following questionnaire.

Food

DO YOU REGULARLY CONSUME THE FOLLOWING?	YES OR NO
Nonorganic foods	
Fatty fish like tuna, swordfish, mahi-mahi, shark, striped bass, and king mackerel	
Foods with corn syrup or high-fructose corn syrup as an ingredient	
Foods with artificial colors, flavors, or sweeteners	
Dairy products	
Fast foods	
Processed foods, which are basically anything you buy in a package that has been dried, frozen, canned, baked, or pasteurized	
Foods made with grains (wheat, oats, rice, barley, etc.)	
Alcohol	
Foods stored in plastic containers	

Environment

DO ANY OF THE FOLLOWING APPLY TO YOUR HOME OR WORK?	YES OR NO
Lawn sprays are used for fertilizers, herbicides, or pesticides	
Insect repellents routinely applied	
Near a nonorganic farm or golf course, or close to an airstrip	

Has potential exposure to gasoline vapors	
Has potential for mold	
Recently renovated, painted, stained, or had new carpeting or wallpaper installed	
Exposes you to car exhaust	
Has an abundance of electronic equipment	
Near a highway, freeway, or other busy major thoroughfare	
Close to power plants, refineries, or oil drilling	
Is a building constructed prior to 1978	

Lifestyle

DO ANY OF THE FOLLOWING APPLY TO YOU?	YES OR NO
Have new furniture or mattresses that are not "green" or organic	
Use personal care products (bodywashes, shampoos, conditioners, lotions, makeup, etc.) that contain ingredients www.ewg.org specifies as toxic	
Wear perfume	
Consume food and beverages that are purchased in plastic (includes water bottles, Keurig cups, and premade microwavable foods, among many others)	
Own a new car	
Take medicines	
Smoke cigarettes or cigars or vape	

DO ANY OF THE FOLLOWING APPLY TO YOU?	YES OR NO
Clean (or have someone clean your home) with bleach, ammonia, or other chemicals www.ewg.org reports as being toxic	
Use air fresheners or burn scented candles	
Use products in aerosol spray cans	
Have your clothes dry-cleaned	
Wear clothes made from synthetic materials	
Work with or regularly around people who manufacture fireworks	
Have amalgam fillings in your teeth	

After completing the questionnaire, you may begin to suspect you need to detox your entire home. If you suspect the problems are at work, well, that's a whole 'nother ball of wax. You'll need to talk with your employer about your concerns there and share what you've learned from this book with them. However, although your hands may be tied at work, your home is your empire. And there are plenty of things you can do to limit your exposure to toxins in your domain.

To get started on detoxing your home, let's think about things that could be off-gassing.

That (Un)Fresh Air Smell

We've already mentioned that you should wash new clothes and let new items have a chance to off-gas before spending any time using them. Some items will take longer than others and, really, the only way you can tell if they are done off-gassing is to give them a good sniff. No smell? They are probably off-gassing much less.

To help new things air out in your home, open your windows (unless your neighbor is tearing down his hundred-year-old, lead-painted house!). Get as much of a cross-breeze as you can. If necessary, you can even get a one-room HEPA air filter to assist with getting those invisible toxins cleaned out of your home.

Sometimes off-gassing can take a few hours, and at other times it can take months. Our daughter took a woodworking class in school where she made a beautiful bedside table that required several coats of lacquer. We are so proud of her! And I'm looking forward to one day having it by my bedside. However, I'm still waiting on being able to bring it inside. It's been off-gassing outdoors for over six months now. See? Off-gassing can take a loooong time.

And, of course, I'm concerned about the kind of fumes she inhaled when painting it.

Many things that off-gas are items from the construction industry, so you'll need to be careful when doing a renovation or building from the ground up.

Build Clean

If you are renovating, having a new home built, or just painting your bathroom, be alert to the products that are used. Often "green" building materials are safe to use, but remember, not everything considered safe for the environment is safe for you. Asbestos, for example, is a naturally occurring mineral, yet you still do not want it or need it in your home! Check the MSDS whenever you can. In particular, here are a few things to be concerned about:

- Paint: as mentioned in my basement story, use no-VOC paint (low-VOC can actually have other harmful chemicals added to it to help lower the smell!)

- Drywall: a lot of drywall is made from something called synthetic gypsum, which has been known to contain mercury, biocides, and other contaminants. Think about all the drywall dust when pieces are cut and sanded! The last thing your body wants is to be breathing in mercury dust! Instead, look for natural, untreated, non-synthetic gypsum.

- Drywall compound / mud and caulk: many of these have high VOCs, so look for low- or non-VOC products

- Plaster: many plasters on the market today contain SVOCs (semi-volatile organic compounds). While that *semi* label may make them sound less harmful, do know they are not harmless *and* they off-gas for the life of the product!

- Insulation: mineral wool is a great option for insulation, as it has zero VOCs

- Glues: many glues contain VOCs and are used to glue down carpets or baseboards

As far as clean building materials go, yes, they can be expensive. But your health is worth it! We recently had a patient who was very sick. She was losing her hair, was extremely fatigued, and had daily headaches. Turns out she was reacting to the foam insulation that her contractor had sprayed inside her walls while renovating her house. The foam put out a tremendous amount of off-gassed chemicals that my patient just couldn't tolerate. Here's the kicker: she had specifically researched this issue and been informed that the spray foam insulation would not off-gas! But it did, and she was super sick. The contractor had to come back and take apart the entire top floor of their home to remedy the situation, during which time she had to move out!

So, on top of the off-gassing, she had to deal with the stress of one renovation after another. I recently spoke with her and learned her foam-removal renovation was finally done. She was back in her home! Her symptoms haven't entirely resolved, but she's continuing to work on detox, and they are diminishing steadily.

Prevent Mold

While I'm on the subject of contractors, don't let them just cover up your walls! Every now and then I see one of those commercials for companies that will cover up your old tubs or showers with a sparkling clean white fiberglass shell, and it scares the hell out of me! The mold will simply fester and grow on whatever they are covering up. And sure, the fiberglass shell looks impermeable when you're standing in front of it, but what's on the other side of that wall? Your bedroom? Your baby's bedroom? Don't risk it. Make them open the walls and get rid of the old stuff!

What to do if you find mold in your home? It's best to hire a professional mold-remediation company to handle the cleanup job for you. But do your due diligence: get referrals and make sure they are one of the best you can find. Not everybody does an equally good job. You want to find someone who will remove anything that even has *potential* for mold. Also, while they are working, be sure to seal off the rest of your house so that the spores don't have the ability to travel and spread. Only when everything is removed and dried out should you start the reconstruction process.

We've spoken so much about mold in this book because it is a pervasive problem and can make you really freaking sick. But it's a problem that sometimes you can't prevent—as when your home is flooded from a pipe break. What you can often prevent is the kind of -cides used in your home: that is, pesticides, herbicides, and fungicides.

Herbicides, Pesticides, and Fungicides

By now, you know you should limit your exposure to pesticides, herbicides, and fungicides. A simple way is just not to spray your lawn with them. There are natural alternatives you can find even in your hardware store. Besides, if you go outside and manually pick the weeds out of your grass and then manually spread seed a couple times during the growing season, not only will you get some exercise, fresh air, and sunshine, you will naturally have a healthier lawn. And for weeds in the cracks of your sidewalk or in areas where no other plants grow, a good spray of vinegar a couple of times on a sunny day will take care of them.

As far as insects go, citronella candles work beautifully to keep mosquitos away—if you do not use them indoors and the scent comes from citronella oil, not from an artificial fragrance. Aside from that, you can plant mosquito-repelling plants like geraniums and lavender. But if you want an added layer of personal protection, tea tree oil makes a great mosquito repellent you can use that will not damage your endocrine system.

Fungicides are their own special category. For years they were considered only mildly irritating to people—like maybe they'd just cause some itchy eyes or runny noses. However, University of North Carolina at Chapel Hill professor Mark Zylka led a research team that discovered some damaging and surprising news about fungicides.

According to their research, common fungicides sprayed on fruits and vegetables cause genetic changes in brain cells in mice. The changes create neurons that are similar to those seen in people who have autism and Alzheimer's disease. So why not play it safe? There are homemade fungicides you can make with baking soda, dish soap, and vegetable oil. Just Google it and you'll find numerous remedies.

Because you can only control pesticides on your property, be aware that anytime you're out in public, you are exposed. And you're eating them in your nonorganic foods! So, do what you can, but don't think you're safe and clean just because your particular home is pesticide-free.

While we're on the subject of pesticides, we can't ignore a major potential avenue of exposure: your pets. I know this is akin to heresy, but...don't let your pets sleep in your bed.

Flea and tick products are toxic! When you put them on Fluffy and Miss Whiskers and then snuggle up to them, you get exposed! And in addition to that, everything that they pick up with their hair from walking around in the world—allergens, chemicals, mold spores—then gets rubbed into your blankets and pillows when they snuggle up with you. (It's also a risk for getting a tick, but that's another book!)

Now that you've gotten rid of the chemicals you put on your yard outside your house, let's look at what you might be exposed to in your house from your cleaning products.

Over and Under the Counters

You can clean quite a bit with vinegar and baking soda, and the best part of it is that neither will hurt you. Then, if you want a pretty smell, use some essential oils mixed into the baking soda. I prefer to use coconut oil–based laundry and cleaning supplies, which work wonders, smell good, and do no harm!

While this is not exactly a cleaning item, it falls under household chemicals: those candles people buy with the "delicious" scents to make their homes smell so good are super toxic! They are scented with petroleum-based ingredients. Would you hover over a barrel of gasoline and breathe in the vapors? No! So stay away from those candles as well as from "air fresheners" you plug in.

Aside from cleaning products, inside your house are plenty of items that could be off-gassing and exposing you to toxins. We've spoken quite a bit about some of these already, but now that your body is clean, let's revisit a few to help you stay clean.

Mattresses

By now you're probably terrified of your mattress. To play it safe, the next time you are in the market for a new mattress, buy one that is organic and *does not contain* a flame retardant (unless you like to smoke in bed—in which case, quit smoking and *then* buy an organic, non-flame-retardant-treated mattress).

It's amazing how easily flame retardants can go through our sheets and into our bodies. Remember my poor mold patient who was exposed to the mold in her school? On her latest toxicity report, she came back showing her mold levels were significantly improving, but she had high levels of flame retardants! Surprised, the first question I asked was if she had recently purchased a new mattress. Yep, she certainly did. And it wasn't an organic one.

In an ideal world, you'd be able to run out and get a new, clean mattress. But because we don't live in an ideal world, let Google be your friend and do some researching. Birch is one company that I found that lists all the certifications about the safety of their products. You can learn about them here: www.birchliving.com/pages/certifications. Birch isn't the only one this good.

There are other companies out there that are just as safe.

If you do buy a clean mattress, you should be able to open it up and sleep on it that night, but you may not be able to. You may still need to off-gas your mattress to release any formaldehyde and other toxins from the textiles. But if you find one that's labeled "shipped stable," that means it was off-gassed at the factory.

Remember, though, that mattresses aren't the only things with flame retardants frequently applied to them. Other items you may be bringing into your home that may have also been treated with flame retardants include upholstered furniture (sofas, chairs, headboards, stools, ottomans, etc.), drapery and other window treatments, and table linens. Read their labels, give them a sniff test (or if you're sensitive, have someone who's less sensitive give them a sniff test) and air out or wash them before using.

While so far we've spoken about household goods and maintenance products, if you've made it this far in the book, you know those aren't the only things you're bringing into the home that could be toxic. So let's look at what we can do about the other "stuff," beginning with our personal care items.

Clean Beauty

We mentioned EWG already a few times. They truly are our favorite go-to for help finding toxin-free products. If you haven't checked out their Skin Deep report, please do so: www.ewg.org.

Also, while we were compiling this book, a new app came onto the market. It's called Think Dirty, and it has a database of ingredients for over 850,000 products. Download it onto your phone, and the next time you are shopping for personal care products, you can scan items with that app and it will tell you all about the potential toxic ingredients in it. Check it out here: www.thinkdirtyapp.com.

From head to toe—shampoo to nail polish—they have just about every product rated for safety. But just in case you can't access it, when you buy anything you put on your skin, look for ingredients you can pronounce. If there are more than three or four syllables in the word—or, heaven forbid, any numbers!—put it back on the shelf and find something else.

Just beware of greenwashing. Greenwashing is when manufacturers use labels and words like *natural* on their products to make them look safer than they really are. Don't fall for a pretty label—read the ingredients.

As we wind up this section on how to be clean in a dirty world, you may be thinking that a lot of money, time, and energy is required to be clean. However, the last trick up our sleeve in this chapter is free and easy! Just kick off those shoes!

Let Your Toes Be Free

I think by now you should be convinced that the world is a very dirty place. And it is! It's also a world where the law of gravity works everywhere. What that means is that all the dirt and toxins in the air eventually find their way to the ground. At that point, it is frequently picked up by the bottoms of shoes.

And you know what? Gravity works inside your home too. So your shoes bring in all those toxins and rub them into the carpeting. Any bare feet that happen to be about get to absorb them. And whatever toxins get kicked up to float around again before resettling become part of your household dust, which easily flies in air currents to be breathed and even eaten.

Taking off your shoes as soon as you come home is probably one of the easiest ways to keep toxins out of your house! But don't forget, if you live in a home built prior to 1978 that hasn't been renovated down to the studs, there's a good chance it contains lead paint. As the home settles, the joints grind up tiny particles, which you end up breathing in and walking on. So if you live in an older home, make sure you wash the floors and even dust the walls regularly!

Whew!

It's exhausting, I know! I wish it weren't, but this is the state of the world we're in. So if you're committed to achieving the best health possible, these are all avenues to take to help get you there.

The good news is that you really can pick and choose what to do and when to do it. Yes, you need to take an all-encompassing look at your life. Get a full inventory of what you are putting in, on, and around your body that could be harmful to you, and then start addressing those areas one at a time.

The thing is, you do need to address them all. Unfortunately, there is no way we could ever prove that there is just one particular toxin that's making you sick and therefore you only need to take this or that particular measure. Toxins build up in your body over time. Eventually a tipping point happens or your rain barrel overflows. So trying to figure out which chemical is the worst for you or the one making you sick isn't going to be effective. That means your best recourse is to clean them all out of your body and then get (and keep) as much out of your environment as possible. Doing that will be the best way for you to look good and feeling freaking fantastic!

Hot Top Tips

1. Freshen your air by opening the windows. Ditch the chemical-based "air fresheners" and candles.

2. Clean with green ingredients.

3. Discover www.ewg.org and use only clean products on your body!

4. Clean up your construction act! One good source we've found is www.greenbuildingsupply.com

5. Don't spray anything toxic on your yard.

6. Buy furniture and bedding that is certified organic.

7. Take off your shoes when you get home.

Conclusion

Congratulations! You made it through what might have been a tough read at times. But now that you've come this far, you're empowered with knowledge and a few tools to help you get started on a new journey of physical health.

We hope we've inspired you to think about your health as something that is *not* predestined but instead is something you *can* control. Yes, *you* are in the driver's seat. And if you make some changes to your lifestyle, you really can live a vibrant, healthy life and feel freaking amazing until you are at least a hundred years old.

Our practice is built around that philosophy. At Five Journeys, we encourage detoxification as only part of the process for achieving and maintaining good health. We don't just create a detox protocol and send our patients back into the world with no other tools. We help them achieve their highest levels of health at any age. To do that, we look at the health of a person across what we consider the five core elements of health: structural, chemical, emotional/mental, social, and spiritual.

Structural

The first core element is all about your bones, joints, ligaments, muscles, and tendons. In theory, they are all built and developed in order to move and perform with ease. When inflammation or deterioration happens, though, that ease is replaced with pain that can lead to a sedentary lifestyle.

By doing a structural analysis of a person's body, we can often discover where the breakdowns are happening and discern the why behind them. Our findings then help us discover the pathways necessary to reverse the inflammation or stop the deterioration.

Your posture is a key element to your structure! Your grandma was right: *stand up straight!* Except now that also refers to *sit up straight* since so many of us sit all day in front of a computer. Because here's the deal: our posture can impact our hormones, specifically our testosterone and cortisol levels. It's true! In studies of posture and the physical positions people take, social psychologist Amy Cuddy and a team of researchers found there was a direct correlation between collapsing your structure (that is, hunching your back and taking up less space) and lowering testosterone and raising cortisol (your stress hormone).[52] Conversely, when you take up more space in "power poses" (think Wonder Woman with feet firmly planted a little more than hip-width apart, fists on hips, back erect), you positively

---

52   D. Carney, A. J. C. Cuddy, and A. Yap, "Power Posing: Brief Nonverbal Displays Affect Neuroendocrine Levels and Risk Tolerance," Psychological Science 21, no. 10 (2010): 1363–1368.

impact your hormone profile (including cortisol). You also positively impact how you are viewed by others.

When discussing your structure with you, Ed and I ask about how frequently you exercise and in what format. While we encourage regular exercise as a key ingredient for your overall general health, our goal is to help you move with ease in whatever form of exercise you enjoy. Right: the kind of exercise you enjoy and not the kind of exercise you feel you need to do because some expert tells you to. If you don't like running, then don't run! Don't think a spinning class is fun? Then don't take one. You don't need to work out to the point where you have 2 percent body fat, nor do you need to run a marathon every day in order to be healthy. In fact, there is such a thing as overexercising, which will cause stress in your body.

But good health requires regular movement and exercise (and don't forget the sweating, which helps you detox!). So it's important to find the right movement for where you are in your life right now. And then, in order for you to continue doing it and receiving the benefits of it, we can address any underlying conditions that might be limiting you in some way.

While we do not subscribe to the belief that everyone must do a particular exercise every day, something we do encourage for all our patients is that they keep in mind how important it is to have a strong core and long spine. Let's face it: it's very hard to be vibrant at age eighty if we're hunched over. Heck, it's hard to be vibrant at any age if we're hunched over! Participating in exercise that strengthens the core and elongates the spine will help prevent that hunching. It will help us to stand or sit up straight. And, hey, we all look good when we have a strong core, right?

Because of that, we love yoga, barre work, and Pilates for their emphasis on core strength as well as on lengthening the spine. The importance of stretching your spine goes beyond "just" keeping us from hunching; it also helps deter spinal compression as we get older—that's when the space between our disks gets smaller. Not only does that make us shorter, but it can cause all sorts of pain, numbness, and other problems in your body. By stretching the spine and doing exercises to strengthen the core several times a week, you can help prevent compression.

Tips for Ensuring You Have Good Structural Health

- Stand up and sit up straight.

- Move your body, every day if possible. Do core and spine-lengthening exercises at least two to three times a week.

- Do deep belly breathing.

- Keep your shoulders down and head up!

Chemical

Your chemical makeup is what the majority of this book has been about. Your body's chemistry is centered around the foods you eat and how well you process and eliminate them. Chemical also involves your hormonal balance, nutrients, minerals, endocrine system, gut function, cardiovascular health, allergies, food sensitivities, and more.

We have a wide range of tests and methods to evaluate your mineral, nutrient, gut, and hormone levels. Once we get that data on you, we can then bring your chemical nature into its natural state of well-being. We can discover allergies and sensitivities, alleviate many other symptoms, and even eradicate diseases and illnesses. Detoxification is just one path to achieve that state. Another way is through proper nutrition.

The clean foods that we discussed in this book are good for everyone, and they will help you achieve a healthy chemical nature. To make it easier to think about food, we like to refer to Michael Pollan's three rules:

1. Eat food.

2. Not too much.

3. Mostly plants.

Of course, once the food comes in, it gets processed, and then the leftovers need to get eliminated. The way you process and digest your food is another great place to find clues about your chemical health. How frequently you poop and what your poop looks like are things we all need to pay attention to. Do you have well-formed brown stools in the shape of a pipe? Great! That's what healthy stool looks like. Anything else likely means there's something hinky in your digestion that should be looked at. Do you think it takes too long for your food to get digested and excreted? Yep, that's worth looking into too. Do you see food particles in your stool? That's also something to evaluate.

It's imperative to have normal, daily bowel movements. If you're not, here are a few things you can try to encourage them to happen.

- Digestive support (taking betaine, pancreatic enzymes, or apple cider vinegar)

- Probiotics

- Spore-based probiotics

- Fermented foods

- Magnesium citrate

- Fiber (both soluble and insoluble)

- Eliminating the top food allergens: gluten, dairy, and sugar

- **Drinking more water**

- **Engaging in vigorous exercise/walking**

- **Doing deep belly breathing and abdominal massage**

Aside from nutrition and digestion, we can look at the quality of your breathing and sleeping as other indicators of your chemical health. I'm sure you know that you breathe in order to get oxygen inside your body, but do you know what oxygen does once it's there? One of the *many* different things it does is help balance the sympathetic and parasympathetic nervous systems to help get us out of the fight-flight-or-freeze mode. Yes, it's oxygen that regulates the balance between stress and relaxation.[53]

Additionally, by breathing deeply, you stimulate the vagus nerve. *Vagus* is Latin for "wandering" and aptly describes this nerve that starts at the brain stem and wanders down both sides of the neck, across the chest, and through the abdomen—connecting your brain with your gut in a roundabout way. The vagus nerve is one of the primary influencers of your parasympathetic system.

---

53 "Deep Breathing to Relieve Acute Stress," UPMC, www.upmc.com/services/healthy-lifestyles/acute-stress/deep-breathing.

Now remember, when you're stressed, one of the things your body does is shut down your digestive system (to get a little technical, it's your sympathetic nervous system that flips the switch). When you can activate your *para*sympathetic system, it will flip the on switch for everything your body shut down in fight-flight-or-freeze mode. But short breaths, or holding your breath, won't activate the parasympathetic system. You need to engage in deep belly breathing. Ever notice how when a baby sleeps, its belly rises and falls with each breath? That's what we mean by deep belly breathing.

In particular, to activate your parasympathetic nervous system, your exhale should be longer than your inhale. That's how you quiet your system and don't jack it up.

An added bonus from this kind of breathing is that it uses the diaphragm and massages the lymph nodes and internal organs, including the gut, which encourages it to move and rev up digestion too. So, by breathing into the belly and making long exhales, you trigger your parasympathetic system *and* stimulate your digestive system, which helps with detoxification.

Oh, and sleep! We've spoken about why it's so important to get good Zs. So you know if you're having trouble there, then you are not detoxing your brain or giving your body a chance to recuperate and rebuild.

Emotional/Mental

We believe your emotional and mental well-being is just as important—if not more important—than your physical well-being. At the time that we are writing this book, COVID-19 has inflated the numbers of people suffering from anxiety and depression to drastic highs. Topping that are fears of economic ruin as our nation struggles to prevent a depression and feelings of isolation because we cannot spend as much time with people in person as we want to. And to make matters worse, many of us are still dealing with the daily stressors we had before the epidemic began: stressors related to family issues, health conditions, job pressure, our children's needs, and on and on and on.

It's heartbreaking to know so many are suffering. But I do know it's possible for us all to heal. And this is where the importance of our brain comes in. For anyone who cannot stop the negative self-talk, who can't sleep from fear and worry, or, on the opposite side, who cannot stay awake because depression is luring them into bed, they *need* to get help healing. It's as imperative for that healing to happen as it is for any physical health improvement to happen.

The good news is there are a multitude of tools available to provide some help. Self-help books, mindfulness classes and retreats, and inspirational books abound. Also, if you pick and choose carefully, there are a multitude of positive, empowering videos on YouTube (there are some that are not so positive and empowering, hence the warning to pick and choose carefully).

And then there are therapists, psychiatrists, and Functional Medicine practitioners, like Ed and me, who understand the connection between our emotions and our physical health. Helping in one area always helps in the other area.

A truly amazing example of the connection between our physical health and our mental and emotional health is my patient, Karen. She was in a very unhappy marriage, so unhappy that it literally made her sick. She was so emotionally locked down that her body just couldn't function properly and it resisted treatment.

It wasn't until she finally divorced her husband—sloughed him off—that her body's resources freed up so she could get well. We were then able to regulate her thyroid. She lost fifteen pounds, and her body was able to detox successfully.

While Karen's story is an inspiring one, don't get the wrong impression. It wasn't the divorce itself that helped Karen heal. It was what she did with her mind as she was going through the divorce and afterward. Just as we have to train our bodies through exercise to be healthy and strong, we have to do the same thing with our mind. We have to train it to think in terms of being happy.

Our minds are programmed to protect us, to survive out in the wild—or inside the mall, or at home in the kitchen, or wherever. We don't consciously think about it, but a large part of our brain is on the constant lookout for threats. That was a handy thing to be going on back in prehistoric times, when there seemed to be a wild animal at the ready to eat us wherever we looked (or should have looked, as the case may be). Although we aren't in that kind of danger anymore, old habits do die hard and, left to their own devices, our brains will keep us in survival mode.

So if we want to surpass surviving and move into thriving, we have to train our brains to think differently. We have to train our minds to slow down enough to choose to listen to the fear-based thoughts or to have the patience to choose a different thought. And you train your mind the same way you train your body: through exercise. The best and most universal training methods for your brain are meditation and prayer.

Here Are Some Tips to Train Your Brain to Improve Your Emotional Health

- Quit relationships that are toxic.

- Watch your language! Negative thoughts are powerful, so work on reframing them to be positive. For example, *I'm never going to be happy* can be reframed as *I'm not happy* yet. Adding *yet* to the end of your sentences can be *extremely* powerful. Try it! *I don't know that yet. I'm not strong enough yet. I'm not fast enough yet.*

- Protect yourself! It's good to be aware of current

> events, but sometimes it's too much, so consider limiting them—especially if they make you anxious!
>
> • Start a meditation practice. Start with at least ten to twenty minutes in the morning. You can choose from a wide variety of apps to get you started. If one doesn't work for you, try another, three others, or even five others before you give up. Remember, meditation is not a destination; it's a practice. So practice every day, whether you want to or not.

Social

The fourth core element of health is concerned with your relationships with friends, your family network, coworkers, or other people you regularly spend time with. In this book, we touched on the importance of eliminating toxic relationships in order to protect your health and promote well-being. But there is more to the social aspect than just your relationships.

To be truly healthy, you must have a sense of belonging to your community. Humans really are social animals, and we all must feel part of a community to achieve optimum wellness.

That community can be your extended family, your work family, your church/synagogue/mosque family, or the group of bird watchers you join the third Sunday of every month. It doesn't matter what your community is, you just need to be part of one. When journalist Dan Buettner first started comparing communities around the world where people regularly lived to be one hundred or older—areas he subsequently named Blue Zones—one of commonalities was a strong sense of community. It is vital that we are part of a strong community, that we have people around us to support us and for us to support in turn. When you can balance a connection to your social group and simultaneously honor your need to be true to yourself, you will also help strengthen your emotional health.

If You Don't Already Have a Strong Social Network, Here Are Some Tips to Help You Start Building One

- Allocate time each week to do something that brings you joy that you can do with others. Do you love to knit? Join a knitting club. Love to read? Join a book club.

- Resolve to call two to three friends a week. Or resolve to communicate with one friend for each: to be seen, to be heard, and to be known (share an experience with).

- Join an organization you appreciate and become a volunteer for them.

- Learn that new skill you've always wanted to by finding a group or class.

Spiritual

Before we discuss the fifth core area, it's important to know that we do not equate being spiritual with adhering to a specific religion or belonging to a church, although we do find both can fulfill the spiritual needs for many people. What we mean by the word *spiritual* is that you have a sense of purpose in your life. That you know your life has meaning and that you are able to connect yourself to that goal.

Some people want us to put off encouraging them to dive into their spirituality. They just want to fix their bodies and get on with their regular business. But if you think about it, having an understanding of what gives your life meaning will propel you to want to take the necessary steps to achieve good health. If someone feels as if there is no purpose to their life, why would they make the effort to eat right? Why would they bother exercising? And seriously, why would they go to the trouble of putting a reverse osmosis filtration on their home's water source?

So sometimes we need to address our spiritual needs first, not last.

**Improving Your Spiritual Health
Means Thinking on
Your Place in the World.**

Tips for doing that:

1. Ask yourself what difference you want to make in this world.

2. Research how to make that happen.

3. Resolve to make a positive difference in another person's life every day, week, or month.

Finding Health

Each of those five core areas is equally important for the creation and maintenance of your overall health. It's by optimally managing each one that we human beings can live vibrant, healthy, happy, and able lives (as well as be interested in intimacy) until we are at least a hundred years old.

To help you figure out where you are on the spectrum of these five pillars, we suggest you review your life and see which areas are most in need of attention right now—and then reach out for help. Often, once someone knows what their main problem is, they find they need to address two or three different core areas to really make a difference in their lives. Which areas will depend on where and how you are experiencing symptoms in your life.

For example, if you are diabetic, nutritionally deficient, or have high blood pressure, then clearly your chemistry needs to be addressed. If you speak negatively about yourself and others, then it may be necessary to give your emotional and mental health some attention.

Whether you address all your issues at one time or begin with one and then pick up another when you're ready is entirely up to you. Please, do what you can and be at peace with where you are. The main thing is to start somewhere and use the tools in this book to help you.

Let's Be Easy

I know you just soaked up a lot of information in this book. To make getting started on your clean life a little easier, there's a checklist in the appendix of everything we spoke about in this book. Pick where you want to begin, and add in the other behaviors and lifestyle changes when you're ready.

You now have tools and resources to get you started on cleaning up your life and your world so you can join me on that poster for clean living. But remember! You do not have to do this alone. You can always contact us at Five Journeys. We do virtual visits with our patients all across the world. Come check out our website, www.fivejourneys.com, and discover what we can do for you.

Also, here's something a little exciting. If you'd like to join a community of like-minded people who are committed to good health and clean bodies, go to our website, www.fivejourneys. com, and check out a virtual detox program we've created where you can join a team of people supporting each other as they go through detox.

Thanks for hanging with us throughout this book! Ed and I truly appreciate your interest, and we hope we can be of service to you as you take your journey to clean health.

The Checklist for Living Clean

Managing Stress

- Get regular sweaty exercise and a good core workout.

- Partake in talk therapy.

- Set yourself up for a good night's sleep.

- Meditate.

- Ask for help—your friends and relatives want you to be healthy too.

- Laugh.

- Be kind to yourself—check for negative self-talk.

- Take a three-day social media detox.

- Get off the grid for a day (or a week if you can swing it!).

- Inventory your relationships. Are any toxic? If so, start working on a plan to distance or divest.

- Identify one thing you can do daily to decrease your stress—and do it!

Food

- Say no to plastics around your food as much as possible— that includes home storage bowls.

- Your municipal water supplier should be able to provide a report on the safety of your drinking water. Find it. Read it. Filter your water if you're concerned!

- Start reading ingredients on food labels.

- Buy organic foods as much as possible.

- Cut out (or at least waaaay back on) sugar.

- Avoid dairy.

- Cut back on alcohol by 50 percent.

- Try to drink only water and green tea (a couple cups of organic coffee, with no milk or sugar, is okay too).

- Eliminate grains or at least those that are glutinous.

- If you're sensitive to mold, avoid these foods:

  * Alcohol made from grains

  * Cheese

  * Coffee

  * Dried fruits and fruit juice

  * Peanut butter

  * Processed meats

  * Wheat, barley, rice, maize

  * Cereals

  * Wine

  * Peanuts and pistachios

  * Leftovers that are older than one day

Personal Care and Lifestyle

- Evaluate where you feel better (or worse). Do your headaches always happen when you're at a particular place? Do you feel worse in certain places than in others?

- Check out www.ewg.org for help finding toxic-free personal care and cleaning products.

- Wash your new clothes before wearing them.

- Find and use an organic dry cleaner.

- Favor clothing made from natural products like cotton, linen, and silk.

- Try to go nontoxic with your lawncare—use vinegar to kill weeds in the cracks of your sidewalks and hand-pull them from the grass.

- Find plants and plant oils that repel mosquitoes and other insects.

- Don't let your pets sleep with you.

- Look for cleaning products made from coconuts or other plants.

- Experiment with using vinegar and baking soda as cleaning agents.

- Open the windows instead of using "air fresheners."

- Take your shoes off when inside your home.

- Buy furniture and mattresses that are certified sustainable or that are shipped stable and do not contain fire retardants.

- Build or renovate green. Use:

    * Non-VOC paint

    * Untreated, natural gypsum drywall

    * Low-VOC drywall compound/mud,
      caulk, and glues

    * Mineral wool insulation

    * Low-VOC glues

Well-Being

- If possible, get a clear family history.

- Get your genes done through Ancestry, 23andMe, or
  another DNA service.

- Run your DNA data through an interpretive program to
  see what your methylation, detox, and other genes put
  you at risk for.

- Inventory your symptoms (and don't just chalk them up
  to aging!).

- Get a Functional Medicine evaluation.

- Get a dry brush and brush your skin to improve
  circulation.

- Spend some time in a sauna or steam bath.

- Try shiatsu, cupping, or other forms of bodywork to improve your circulation.

- Test your water and air at home (and try to get it done at work too!).

- Quit drinking from single-use plastic bottles.

- Use good posture—shoulders back, head up.

- Engage in exercise that strengthens your core and elongates your spine.

- Get regular physical movement.

- Do deep belly breathing.

- Pay attention to your bowel movements—get help if they are not healthy.

- Get good sleep.

- Allocate time each week to do something that brings you joy that you can do with others. Do you love to knit? Join a knitting club. Love to read? Join a book club.

- Resolve to call two to three friends a week. Or resolve to communicate with one friend for each: to be seen, to be heard, and to be known (share an experience with).

- Join an organization you appreciate and become a volunteer for them.

- Learn that new skill you've always wanted to learn by finding a group or class.

- Ask yourself what difference you want to make in this world. Research how to make that happen.

Toxin Sources and What to Do

What's not included in this list is what we've covered extensively in the book—mycotoxins from mold, pesticides, herbicides, fungicides, and heavy metals—so keep those in mind!

SUBSTANCE	SOURCES	ASSOCIATED CLINICAL ISSUES	REMOVAL	PREVENTION
2-Hydro-xyisobutyric Acid (2HIB)	Gasoline additives derived from MTBE/ETBE; comes from groundwater contamination, inhalation, or skin exposure	Hepatic, kidney, and central nervous system (CNS) toxicity, neurotoxicity, cancer in animals	Sauna therapy Niacin Glutathione N Acetyl Cysteine	

SUBSTANCE	SOURCES	ASSOCIATED CLINICAL ISSUES	REMOVAL	PREVENTION
Mono-ethylphthalate (MEP)	Diethylpthalates; comes from bath/beauty products, cosmetics, perfumes, pharmaceuticals, insect repellants, adhesives, inks, varnishes	Reproductive damage, depressed leukocyte function, impedes blood coagulation, lowers testosterone	Sauna therapy Niacin Glutathione NAC	
2-3-4 methyl-hippuric acid	Derived from xylene; found in paints, lacquers, pesticides, cleaning fluids, fuel, exhaust, perfumes, insect repellants	Nausea, vomiting, dizziness, CNS depression, death	Niacin Glycine Glutathione NAC	
Phenyl-glyoxylic acid (PGO)	Derived from styrene/ethyl-benzene; found in car exhaust, building materials, plastics, food packaging materials	Concentration issues, fatigue, nausea, muscle weakness, irritates mucous membranes of nose/mouth/eyes	Sauna therapy Glutathione NAC	Use glass instead of plastic containers.
N-acetyl-phenyl-cysteine (NAP)	Derived from benzene; found in mechanical processes, combustion, car exhaust, cigarettes	Nausea, vomiting, dizziness, CNS depression, death, lack of coordination	Sauna therapy Niacin Glutathione NAC	

SUBSTANCE	SOURCES	ASSOCIATED CLINICAL ISSUES	REMOVAL	PREVENTION
N-acetyl (2-cyanoethyl) cysteine (NACE)	Derived from acrylonitrile; found in production of acrylic resins, fiber, and rubber; also found in cigarette/ tobacco smoke	Headaches, nausea, dizzi- ness, fatigue, chest pains; classified as a carcinogen by European Union	Glutathione NAC	
Perchlo- roethylene (PERc)	Derived from perchlorate; found in rocket fuel, missiles, flares, fireworks, explosives, fertil- izers, bleach; also found in water supply and foods (cow's milk, eggs, vege- tables, fruit)	Disrupts the thyroid; classified as a carcin- ogen by EPA	Use a reverse osmo- sis water filtra- tion system to remove perchlorates from water.	Use a reverse osmosis water filtra- tion system to remove perchlorates from water.
Diphenyl phosphate (DPP)	Derived from triphenyl phosphate (flame retardant); found in plastics, nail polish, resins, elec- tronic equipment	Linked to endo- crine disruption, reproductive and developmen- tal problems	Removed from body via the glucuronos- yltransferase enzymes (phase 2 liver)	Avoid PVC piping, rubber, pigments and paints.

SUBSTANCE	SOURCES	ASSOCIATED CLINICAL ISSUES	REMOVAL	PREVENTION
2-hydroxyethyl mercapturic (HEMA)	Derived from ethylene oxide, halopropane, vinyl chloride; found in agrochemicals, detergents, pharmaceuticals, personal care products, aerosol propellants	Autism, breast cancer, leukemia, CNS depression, nausea, headaches, dizziness, thrombocytopenia, liver damage, death; classified as a carcinogen by multiple agencies	Infrared sauna therapy Niacin B12 therapy Glutathione	Eliminate use of all plastic containers, especially for warm/heated foods/drinks.
N-acetyl (propyl) cysteine (NAPR)	Derived from 1-bromopropane; found in metal cleaning, dry cleaning, foam, gluing	Neurological and reproductive toxin; causes sensory and motor deficits, decreased cognitive impairment, headaches	Glutathione NAC	Evaluate environment to determine source of exposure.
N-Acetyl (2,Hydroxypropl) Cysteine (NAHP)	Derived from propylene oxide; found in plastics and fumigants along with lubricants, surfactants, oil demulsifiers	Probable carcinogen; found in food additives, insecticides, herbicides, microbicides, fungicides, miticides; may cause corneal burns, dermatitis, DNA damage	Glutathione NAC	

SUBSTANCE	SOURCES	ASSOCIATED CLINICAL ISSUES	REMOVAL	PREVENTION
N-acetyl-S-(2-carba-moylethyl) cysteine (NAE)	Derived from acrylamide; found in plastics, food packaging, water treatment, dyes, cosmetics, foods containing asparagine cooked at high temps (potato chips) as well as asparagus, beef, fish, potatoes, nuts, seeds, legumes	Causes neurological damage, raises cancer risk, causes muscular atrophy; carcinogenic properties	Glutathione NAC	
N-acetyl (3,4-dihy-droxybutyl) cysteine (NADB)	Derived from 1,3-butadiene; used in production of synthetic rubber (think: tires)	Known carcinogen; increases risk of cardiovascular disease	Glutathione NAC	Avoid playgrounds and athletic fields made with ground-up tires.

SUBSTANCE	SOURCES	ASSOCIATED CLINICAL ISSUES	REMOVAL	PREVENTION
				Eat organic foods to reduce exposure. Avoid lice shampoo, pet flea collars, and flea spray.
Diethyl phosphate/ dimethyl phosphate (DEP/DMP)	Derived from organophosphates; found in pesticide formulations	Overstimulates nerve cells, leading to sweating, overstimulation, diarrhea, aggression, and depression/suicide; children of exposed mothers have increased risk of pervasive developmental disorder	Acute exposure treated with atropine/ pralidoxime. Non-acute remedy: sauna treatment	Avoid spraying pesticides in house or garden; don't live near agricultural areas or golf courses; stay indoors if insecticides are being sprayed.
2,4-dichlorophenoxyacetic acid	Herbicide that was part of Agent Orange; found in agriculture, genetically modified foods, weed killer	Causes neuritis, weakness, abdominal pain, nausea, headaches, dizziness, seizures, brain damage; also a powerful endocrine disruptor; linked to immune system damage, birth defects, and reproductive issues	Sauna treatment Niacin supplementation Vitamin B12 therapy Glutathione NAC	Remove exposures.

SUBSTANCE	SOURCES	ASSOCIATED CLINICAL ISSUES	REMOVAL	PREVENTION
3-hydroxy-propylmer-capturic acid (3-HPMA)	Derived from acrolein; found in environmental pollutants, herbicides, cigarettes, gasoline and oil, fried foods, cigarette smoke, auto exhaust	Associated with diabetes and insulin resistance; plays a role in spinal cord injury, MS, Alzheimer's disease, cardio-vascular disease, diabetes, neuro-, hepato-, nephro-toxicity; causes oxidative stress, mitochondrial disruption, immune dysfunction	NAC Glutathione	

Acknowledgments

When we began writing this book, we knew it would be time-consuming. We knew it wouldn't be the easiest thing we've ever done. And we knew we couldn't do it without the support from everyone in our lives, especially from our children. Thank you, Gabriella, Arianna, Etan, and Rafaella. Each one of you is a complete and total gift! We are *so* lucky to be your parents. Thanks for being born to us and for being so supportive of our work!

We also want to thank our parents: Gail, Anna, Marshall, and Ron. It's really true: it takes a village. We are beyond grateful that you are part of ours! We could not do any of this without you. And our appreciation extends to Lenny Levitan, in memory of him and his passion for life, which serves as a constant inspiration for us.

In addition to our parents, we have been blessed to have some amazing mentors and coaches helping us, including Ramdass Rao, Kathy Clabby, and Diane Desroche. Thank you! We're all about leveling up, and you have been instrumental in assisting us with getting there (then leveling up again!).

Part of leveling up in the book was in ensuring our science is backed up by data. For that, we thank our scientific advisor, John Bagnulo, MPH, PhD, for the research he did to help make this book a reality. Drama? You bet. Inaccurate? Hard no. Thanks for making sure the science is accurate!

To our team at Five Journeys: each of you has been instrumental in ensuring our practice flows smoothly. Thanks for taking care of the details so we could write this book!

What good can a book do if no one knows about it? None! So we thank Amanda Klotz and Renee and Andrew Newland of the FMM team. Thank you for jumping in to assist us every time we needed you.

We also thank those who made the actual book possible, our team at Scribe Media: Kayla Sokol, Lisa Shiroff, Barbara Boyd, Rachael Brandenberg, and Sheila Parr. From writing to visuals, you've each done such a fabulous job. We are so grateful! This book would not have been written without you.

Of course, we can't forget to thank our patients. We wish we could name each and every one of you, but the book spine cannot get that big. Please know we really are in this with you. Thank you for your generosity, for your trust, and for being amazing sources of cool new treatments!

Before we go, we also must thank Dr. Mark Hyman, Mel Robbins, and Len Schlesinger for believing in us, pre-reading our book, and saying such nice things about it!

About the Authors

Husband-and-wife team Wendie Trubow and Ed Levitan are physicians and Functional Medicine practitioners with more than thirty-five years of combined experience in the medical field. Their first Functional Medicine practice became the largest in the nation during its time. Eight years later, they launched their membership-based wellness organization, Five Journeys, where they focus on the integration of five core areas of health to create comprehensive, individualized wellness plans for their members.

Ed and Wendie live in the Boston area with their four kids, two cats, nine chickens, and, of course, their sauna, the newest addition to their family!

CPSIA information can be obtained
at www.ICGtesting.com
Printed in the USA
JSHW080152220323
39290JS00001B/66